SERIOLOGICAL DIAGNOSIS OF CERTAIN HUMAN, ANIMAL AND PLANT DISEASES

Edited by **Moslih Al-Moslih**

Serological Diagnosis of Certain Human, Animal and Plant Diseases
Edited by Moslih Al-Moslih

Published by InTech
Janeza Trdine 9, 51000 Rijeka, Croatia

Publishing Process Manager Iva Simcic

Technical Editor Teodora Smiljanic

Cover Designer InTech Design Team

Additional hard copies can be obtained from orders@intechopen.com

Serological Diagnosis of Certain Human, Animal and Plant Diseases,
Edited by Moslih Al-Moslih
p. cm.
ISBN 978-953-51-0370-7

For EU product safety concerns:
IN TECH d.o.o., Prolaz Marije Krucifikse Kozulić 3, 51000 Rijeka, Croatia,
info@intechopen.com or visit our website at intechopen.com.

Meet the editor

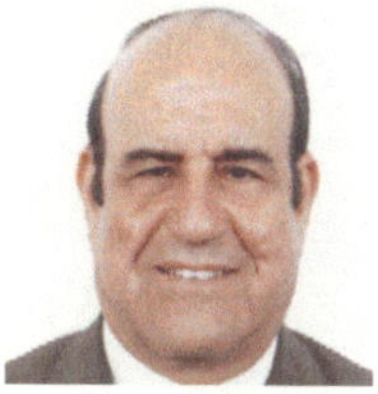

Dr Moslih Al-Moslih received his PhD (1972) in medical microbiology from the University of Nebraska, Medical Center, Omaha, Nebraska, USA. He went on to work as assistant professor in the same department at Nebraska Medical Center. He taught two courses in microbiology: one for undergraduate medical students and the other course for graduate students. He also supervised medical lab diagnosis and a research project related to EBV and Burkitt's lymphoma using the transfection method to explore transformation by EB virus in cell culture. He was a member of the American Society for Microbiology (ASM) and the International Society for Infectious Diseases (ISID) and FISBT. Professor Al-Moslih has published more than 84 scientific papers in different abstracted, refereed and indexed journals and four books in microbiology for third year medical students. Most of these papers were in the area of infectious and molecular diseases. He has worked as consultant for several institutes and government agencies on a national and international level.

Contents

Preface

In this book we have the great privilege to coordinate a special overview of the laboratory diagnoses of certain infectious disease agents. The chapters have been written by some of the gifted scientists who are experts in this field. The book deals with some of the aspects of infectious diseases caused by bacteria, viruses, parasites and protozoa as well as autoimmune disease. Microbiologists, infectious disease specialists, and immunologistall contributed to this volume. Indeed, our main goal was to cover a broad range of the characteristics of the infectious diseases caused by different microorganisms and to provide current, state-of-the-art guidelines on serological laboratory diagnosis.

In the last part of this volume, an autoimmune disease is addressed in the form of a diagnostic method.

We sincerely hope that this book will be of help and interest to all infectious disease specialists and healthcare providers involved in the diagnosis and care of patients as well as plants.

Moslih Al-Moslih
Adjunct Professor, Infectious Disease Section,
Dept of Pediatrics, College of Medicine,
University of Colorado, Denver,
USA

Part 1

Serological Diagnosis of Bacterial Diseases

1

Helicobacter pylori Infection and Undiagnosed Dyspepsia in Dyspeptic Populations Under 45 of Age Tested by ELISA, Urease Breath Test and Helicotest

Małgorzata Palka
Department of Family Medicine,
Jagiellonian University Medical College, Kraków,
Poland

1. Introduction

1.1 *Helicobacter pylori* infection

One-half of the world's population is infected with *Helicobacter pylori (H. pylori),* a gram negative bacterium which is responsible for various major upper digestive tract diseases. *H. pylori* is one of the most common bacterial pathogens in humans, who are the only known host of *H. pylori* The human stomach is considered the reservoir of this bacteria.

H. pylori has been cultured from saliva, dental plaque, vomitus, and diarrheal stool demonstrating that the bacterium is potentially transmissible by these routes. The main route of transmission is not yet clearly understood.

H. pylori transmission is believed to be mainly familial, and there is epidemiological evidence that shows that the infection spreads via person-to-person contact (14). Moreover, potential reservoirs of bacterium are through to be animals who are in close contacts with humans: cats, dogs, pigs, and birds. There is also the hypothesis that the most predominant mode of transmission is mother-to-child via contact with regurgitated gastric juice from the mother's mouth. The most common accepted routes of transmission are fecal-oral in developing countries, and gastro-oral route in developed countries. There are many risk factors for *H. pylori* infection including: overpopulation/congested houses, family sizes, unsafe sources of water, and low socioeconomic status (17).

The common risk factors for *H. pylori* infection is:

- crowding
- low level of personal hygiene
- low family income
- unclean drinking water
- lack of toilet facilities during childhood
- low educational level
- previous gastrointestinal endoscopy

H. pylori infection is recognized as a worldwide problem as it causes chronic gastritis, peptic ulcer disease, and Mucosa-Associated Lymphoid Tissue lymphoma. *H. pylori* is also a major risk factor for gastric cancer. The global burden of gastric cancer is considerable but varies in different countries, with more than 70% of cases occurring in developing countries especially in Eastern Asia. In 2008, it was estimated that there would be just under one million new cases of stomach cancer (Tab.1) Stomach cancer accounts for 7.8% of the all total cancers worldwide, and it is currently the fourth most common malignancy in the world, behind lung cancer, breast cancer, and colon cancer. Stomach cancer is more common in men (640 000) than in women (348 000), and half of the world's stomach cancers occur in Eastern Asia and China. The highest mortality rates are estimated in Eastern Asia (28.1 per 100,000 in men, 13.0 per 100,000 in women), and the lowest in Northern America (2.8 and 1.5, respectively). High mortality rates are present in both sexes in Europe, and in Central and South America.

Estimated numbers (thousands)	**Men**		**Women**		**Both sexes**	
	Cases	**Deaths**	**Cases**	**Deaths**	**Cases**	**Deaths**
World	640	463	348	273	988	736
More developed regions	173	110	101	70	274	180
Less developed regions	467	353	246	202	713	55
China	315	231	148	121	463	352
European Union (EU-27)	50	37	32	24	82	61

Globocan 2008

Table 1. Stomach Cancer Incidence and Mortality Worldwide

The prevalence of *H. pylori* ranges from <10-20% in the USA, 40% in Germany, and 30-40% in England to more than 70% in Eastern Europe or even up to 90% Asia and Africa. The percentile of infection is also higher in rural areas than in big cities (5).

There are differences in *H. pylori* prevalence between high and low-income countries because *H. pylori* infection is strongly related to economic conditions (17). *H. pylori* incidence also increases with age largely due to the birth cohort effects. The children are re-infected more frequently than adults and because the close contact between young children, especially among siblings and children under the age of 5. In developing countries infection occurs in the first years of life and increases successively involving almost 90% of the 50-year-olds. In developed countries it affects only a small percentage of children below 10 years of age and does not exceed 40% in adults. It has been suggested that treating infected children reduces the transmission of infection and ultimately reduces the gastric cancer in adults, but the role of potential *H. pylori* eradication for the prevention of gastric cancer is still unknown.

The effects of *H. pylori* infection on human gastric physiology are complex. Presence of the bacteria induces chronic inflammation via the release of chemokines and cytokines. *H. pylori* infection also stimulates the human immune system, causing T and B lymphocytes, along with neutrophils and monocytes to produce antibodies (Ig G and IgA) and cytokines (TNF alpha, interleukin). This immune response is unable to eliminate the pathogen and leads to persistent gastric mucosal damage as more neutrophils, lymphocytes, and plasma cells are recruited to chronic inflammatory sites (Tab.2).

Activation of limphocyte	**Stimulation of neutrophile and monocyte**
• Lymphocyte B (↑Ig G, ↑IgA) in human blood	• ↑Histamine
• Lymphocyte T (IL-2,IL-8, TNF alfa)	• ↑ Interleukin (IL-1,IL-6, IL-8)
	• ↑ TNF alfa
	• ↑ Interferon
	• ↑ Prostoglandin E2

Table 2. The human immune system response to *H. pylori* infection

The virulence of the bacteria depends on the presence of the cag pathogenicity island which is a 35-40 kb genomic fragment containing 29 genes. The cagA protein is a well-known virulence marker encoded by the cagA gene. The presence of this gene has been associated with both duodenal ulcers and gastric cancer. CagA is phosphorylated and binds to SHP-2 tyrosine phosphatase and induces the intracellular signaling processes.

Another virulence marker is 95-kd vacuolating cytotoxin VacA which is related to the cag pathogenicity island. The VacA toxin opens the membrane channels of gastric epithelial cells to give the bacteria nutrients, and the mitochondrial membrane releases cytochrome c to induce apoptosis.

The *H. pylori* infection can be diagnosed by invasive and noninvasive testing (Tab.3). "Test and treat strategy" everywhere in *H. pylori* infection is recommended for patients with uninvestigated persistent dyspepsia less than 45, 50 or 55 years depending on country's guidelines without any alarm features (24, 25, 26). The "test and treat strategy" is based on non-invasive testing of *H. pylori* infection.

H. pylori diagnostic tests	
Invasive	**Non-invasive**
Gastroscopy • standard videoendoscopy • high magnifying endoscopy • chromoendoscopy	**Serology** • near patient tests (HelicoTest) • ELISA
Rapid urease test (CLO test)	**UBT test C13, C14**
Histology (Giemsa staining)	**HP stool antigen test (HPSA)** • polyclonal antibody-based ELISA • monoclonal antibody -based ELISA
Microbiology Culture	**Gastropanel** • *H. pylori* antibodies • Pepsinogen I, II • Gastrin 17

Table 3. Diagnostic modalities of *H. pylori* infection

1.2 Functional dyspepsia

The detection of current *H. pylori* infection is becoming more important clinically, especially in young patients, because the eradication of infection is likely to affect the natural course of the disease and modify the risk of gastric cancer. Early detection and eradication of *H. pylori* in the population will decrease major upper tract organic diseases as well (13).

Strategies to improve the management of *H. pylori* infection in the dyspeptic population with upper gastrointestinal symptoms have been shown to reduce mortality in the population caused by *H. pylori* infection. It is good to note that there is still more research needed regarding serology tests in young dyspeptic patients.

The Maastricht III-2005 Consensus report recommended serology as an alternative option for countries with a high prevalence of *H. pylori* infection (19, 20). The two serology tests that are most often used are the ELISA test and the near patients tests. The serology tests have the lowest cost per correct diagnosis at low (30%), intermediate (60%), and high prevalence (90%) of *H. pylori* infection but their diagnostic accuracy is lower than other noninvasive tests. The Urea Breath Test (UBT) is more costly, more time consuming, and needs special preparation by the patient, such as fasting and cessation of antibiotics, proton pump inhibitors (PPI), and H_2 blockers. The doctors who care for undiagnosed dyspeptic patients need to be aware of the value of these serology tests in young patients.

2. Dyspepsia and gastrointestinal symptoms

Gastrointestinal symptoms are common, with up to one in three people in population-based studies reporting symptoms from the gastrointestinal tract (Tab.4). Research published in 2008 in Sweden has shown a prevalence of symptoms from upper and lower gastrointestinal tract in adult population study even up to 60%. Symptom flux over time provides primary care physicians with a significant workload.

Gastrointestinal symptoms	Pain modalities
1. Acid regurgitation	1. Aching
2. Belching	2. Butterflies
3. Burning feeling rising from the stomach up towards the neck	3. Burning sensation
	4. Cramp
4. Dysphagia	5. Colic
5. Early satiety	6. Gripes
6. Heartburn	7. Pain
7. Nausea	8. Tenderness
8. Loss of appetite	9. Twinge
9. Loss of weight	10. Stitch
10. Pain behind the breast bone	11. Sinking feeling
11. Uncomfortable feeling of fullness	
12. Vomiting (recurrent)	

Table 4. The 12 general upper gastrointestinal symptoms from Carlsson & Drossman.
11 abdominal discomfort or pain modalities.

Gastrointestinal symptoms have been grouped into several entities (Fig.2). Depending on the symptoms profile, dyspeptic symptoms ranged from 15-40% in the population, reflux symptoms 15-25%, and irritable bowel symptoms 10-20%. About 14% of all patients will have dyspeptic, reflux, and irritable bowel symptoms when they are presenting in the primary care setting.

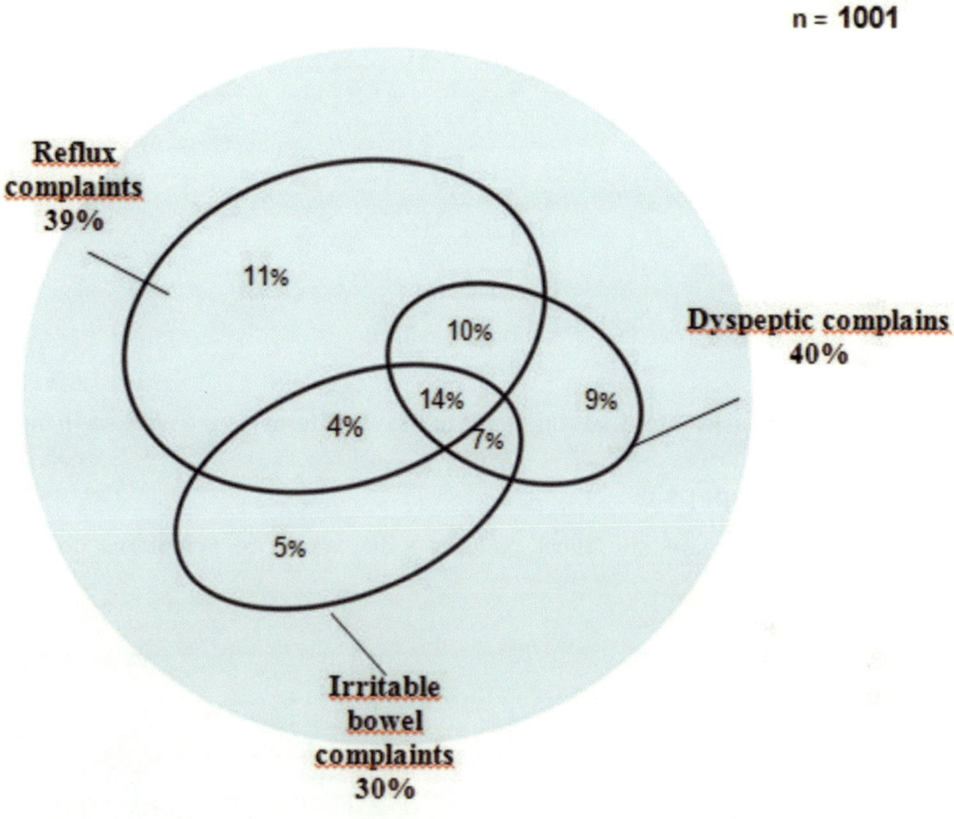

Fig. 2. The prevalence of reflux, dyspeptic and irritable bowel complaints in the general population.

Data was collected from two neighboring communities in Northern Sweden, Kalix and Haparanda, with 18,408 and 10,580 inhabitants, respectively (Kalixandra Study) has showed that most gastrointestinal complaints classified as reflux, dyspeptic, or irritable bowel complaints lasts over 6 month.

The short-term fluctuation of gastrointestinal symptoms in the general population is a fact (Fig.3). Reflux complaints are slightly more stable in comparison to the dyspeptic symptoms or irritable bowel complaints. During times of stress and emotional problems dyspeptic problems can be more severe and cause more problems for the patient, but only a fraction of sufferers will seek medical care (4). It is important to remember that troublesome gastrointestinal complaints remained present in approximately 90% of subjects in all symptoms groups if not diagnosed and treated.

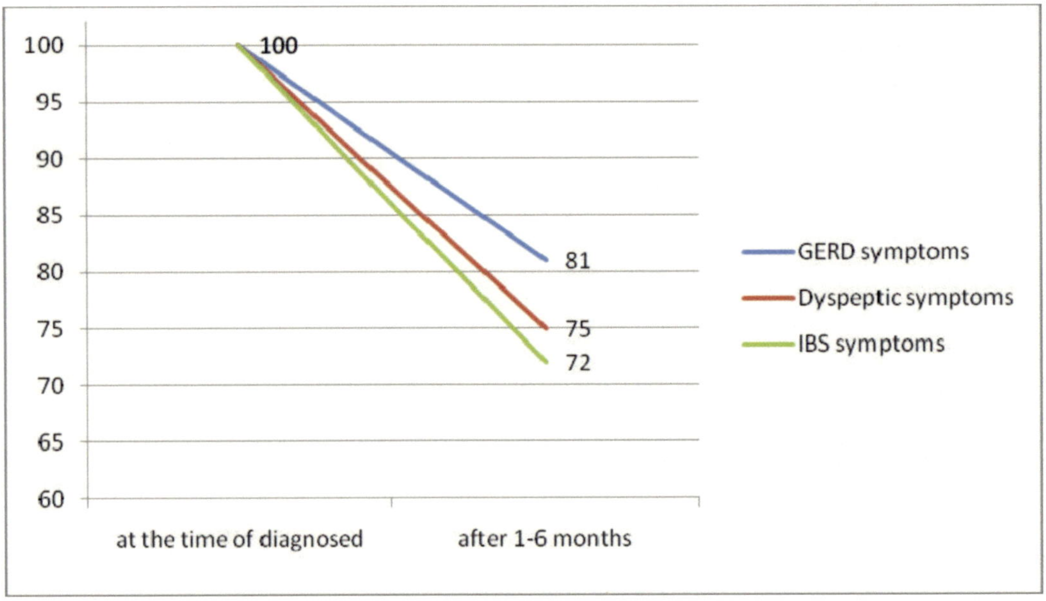

Fig. 3. Fluctuation of gastrointestinal complains in the short term from 4 weeks to 6 months.

3. Undiagnosed dyspepsia

Dyspepsia is very common and most patients will experience symptoms occasionally (Fig.4).

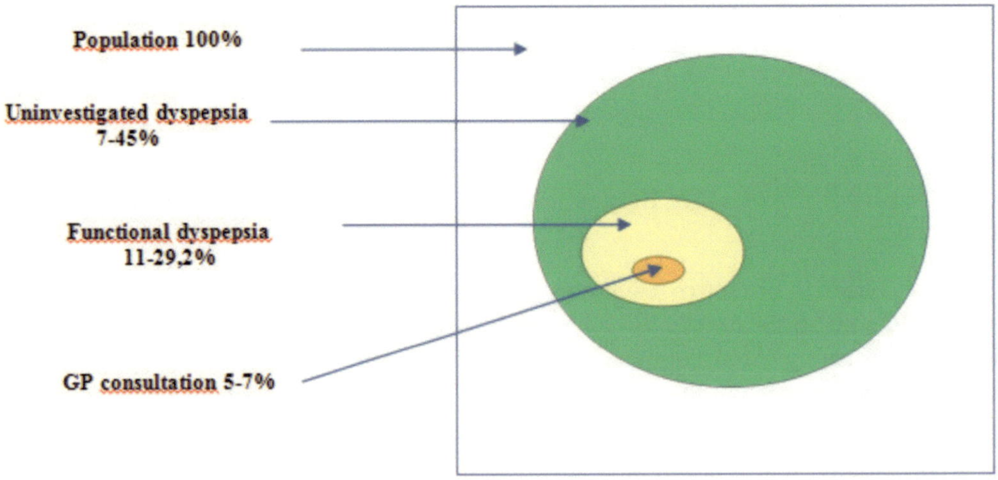

Fig. 4. Prevalence of dyspepsia in the community.

If the symptoms are chronic and recurrent medical management is needed. If the patients have symptoms occurring more than twice a week or lasting for over 4 weeks medical help is needed because of the major decrease in quality of life (2).

The life impairment and impact of undiagnosed dyspepsia on health-related quality of life (HRQOL) is significantly lower in dyspeptic patients than in healthy controls (0,85+/-0,17 vs 0,95+/-0,12) p<0,0001 (15).

Dyspepsia is diagnosed as a syndrome consisting of pain or discomfort centered in the upper abdomen (epigastric pain), burning, fullness, discomfort, early satiety, nausea, vomiting, and belching.

Many patients with undiagnosed dyspepsia are usually young and there is overlap of symptoms and findings in performed investigations regarding to most functional symptoms like Irritable Bowel Syndrome or Functional Heartburn (9).

If alarm symptoms occur in patients with undiagnosed dyspepsia, upper gastroscopy is needed (Tab.5).

• Signs and symptoms of upper gastrointestinal bleeding
• Unexplained anemia
• Unexplained weight loss
• Progressive dysphagia
• Recurrent vomiting
• Progression of symptoms
• Previous gastric surgery
• Family history of gastrointestinal cancer
• <45,50, or 55 years of age (depending on country)

Table 5. Alarm symptoms for uninvestigated dyspepsia and indications for upper gastrointestinal endoscopy.

The epidemiology of dyspepsia can influence of many factors such as: cultural differences in reporting of symptoms of dyspepsia, socio-economic status, cigarette smoking, *H. pylori* infection, use of non-steroidal anti-inflammatory drugs, and alcohol consumption (Tab.6).

• Main Risk Factors:	• Odds Ratio
• *H. pylori* infection	• OR 1,21 (CI;1,03-1,42)
• Cigarette smoking 20/day	• OR 1,55 (CI;1,29-1,86)
• Unemployment	• OR 2,18 (CI2,86-2,56)
• Daily use of ASA/NSAID	• OR 2,33 (CL;1,72-3,15)
• Others: Alcohol consumption, social status, life style factors, level of education	

Table 6. Risk factors for dyspepsia in a general population a total 10 007 aged 40-64 years.

Research has shown that patients profiles and risk factors are important in the management of dyspepsia, and its role is increasing with the patients age. Common use of non-steroidal anti-inflammatory drugs, high prevalence of *H. pylori* infection in many countries, and the increasing prevalence of smoking in the young population make dyspepsia a very common ailment (31).

Initial management with prompt endoscopy slightly more effective (3,7,8) compared to the "test and treat" approach for inducing resolution of symptoms, but is not as cost effective as the "test and treat" strategy (Tab.7).

Outcomes	RRR (CI)
Presence of symptoms	5% (1 to 8) significant difference favours for endoscopy
	Standardised mean difference (95% CI)
Total dyspepsia symptoms score	-0,11 (-028 to 0,07)
	Weighted mean difference (CI)
Additional cost of prompt endoscopy (US dollars)	$389 (276-502) significant differences favour "test and treat strategy"

Table 7. Initial management of dyspepsia with prompt endoscopy v "test and treat" strategy at 12 month.

There is an overlap of symptoms and finding structural abnormalities in upper endoscopy, however about 60% of all endoscopies performed will not find any structural changes in upper digestive track (Fig.5).

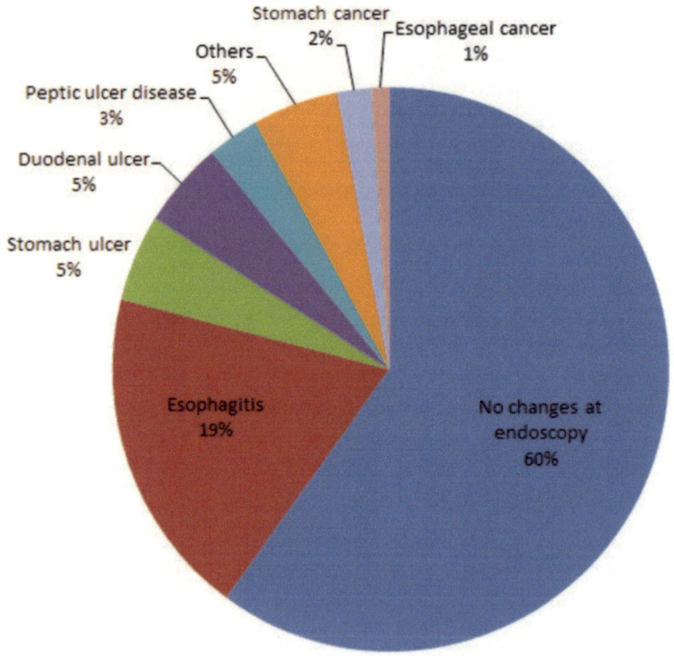

Fig. 5. Abnormal finding at upper digestive track during performing gastroscopy.

40% of all patients with dyspeptic complaints will have some small mucosal changes in upper gastrointestinal tract. Ford et al. provide the first meta-analysis of individual patients of 5 management trials. Their results strongly support the "test and treat" strategy in terms of cost effectiveness. The prevalence of organic dyspepsia as classified by endoscopy increased with the patient's age (23). A proportion of patients have an underlying organic cause for their symptoms such as peptic ulcer disease or reflux esophagitis. However, only 3% of people in the population-based study were found to have an organic disease diagnosed in the general health care system.

Peptic ulcer was found in only 3.9% of all subjects with upper abdominal symptoms in population based study by Bernersen et al. Aro et al. found that 4.1% of the subjects have peptic ulcers and minority of those with gastroesophageal reflux disease were found to have esophagitis on endoscopy which still is the most commonly found change on this procedures (29).

There is great debate in the medical community about whether gastrointestinal symptoms in the general population should be regarded as a disease or not. Many cases of epigastric pain are diagnosed as functional dyspepsia (FD) without any organic changes found in upper endoscopy. FD can be diagnosed if the symptoms are chronic and not caused by another organic, systemic, or metabolic disease. Many of those with dyspeptic symptoms will have functional dyspepsia, gastrointestinal motor abnormalities, or altered visceral sensation. FD can be considered as bio-psychological disorder causing a dysregulation of the brain-gut axis (1).

A meta-analysis of 9 trials evaluating a total of 2541 patients with FD found a modest but significant benefit to *H. pylori* eradication treatment at 12 months. According to the analysis the mean response rate to placebo at 1 year was 28% (range 7-51%) and the mean response rate to *H. pylori* eradication 36% (range 21-58%). Many researchers thinks that eradication *H. pylori* might be a cost-effective intervention for FD.

4. The aim of the study

1. The main aim of the study was to compare the accuracy of serology tests (ELISA, HelicoTest) with the benchmark UBT in the detection of *H. pylori* infection in young dyspeptic patients age 20-45 who presented with chronic dyspeptic symptoms over 6 months at the primary care setting.
2. The additional aims of the study determine whether a correlation existed between the level of Ig G antibodies and positive UBT test.

5. Material and methods

The study was conducted from 2004-2006 in the primary care setting in Cracow. Each of the enrolled patients underwent the following procedures:

- Detailed history
- Physical examination
- C13 Urease UBT test
- Serological ELISA-DPC test
- HelicoTest - a rapid test for quick detection of IgG antibodies
- Epidemiological questionnaire using the Glasgow Dyspepsia Severity Score (GDSS) which assesses dyspepsia symptoms (10).

The most frequent symptoms of dyspeptic patients were: epigastric pain, upper abdominal discomfort before and after a meal, and dysmotility-related symptoms (bloating, nausea, belching, occasional heartburn). The study was approved by the Ethics Committee of the Jagiellonian University, and all participants gave written informed consent. The gold standard of diagnosis of *H. pylori* infection was based on a positive UBT test. Patients with alarm symptoms were not included into the study.

Exclusion criteria included: weight loss, anaemia, hematemesis, melena, abdominal tumor, use of non-steroidal anti-inflammatory drugs, use of antibiotics or ranitidine bismuth citrate four weeks prior to the investigation, use of PPI two weeks and H_2 blockers 48 hours prior to investigation.

Statistical analysis was carried out using the STATISTICA and SAS programs. The agreement of the tests was assessed by three criteria: the percentage of incompatible results, the value of the kappa coefficient, and McNemara's test for related dichotomous variables. $P<0.05$ was considered statistically significant. Distinguishing a positive or a negative *H. pylori* result was objective in UBT and positive ELISA was considered at the level of 1.00 U/ml.

6. Results

The study group consisted of 159 patients. Patients characteristics are shown in (Tab.8).

Study group	Mean age	Sex		Smokers	Non smokers
		Female	Men		
159 patients	34,79	(73,6%)	(26,4%)	(16,4%)	(83,6%)

Table 8. The study patient groups' characteristics

The men had higher level of Ig G antibodies than women see tab.9.

Group [U/ml]	Sex [U/ml]	
	Female	Men
study [1,83]	1,76	2,02

Table 9. The mean level of Ig G antibodies depending on the patient's sex.

The majority of patients have moderate symptoms. Acute symptoms were only found in a minority of patients (Tab.10,11,12). The most common symptoms from the tested population are shown in the following tables.

Study group 159	Type of dyspeptic symptoms (%)			
	Severe	Moderate	Mild	Not specific
	18.2	59.8	17	5.0

Table 10. Severity of symptoms in the study population.

Study group (%)					
Upper abdominal pain	**Heartburn**	**Discomfort in upper area**	**Belching**	**Nausea**	**Flatulence**
76,1	62,2	68,5	50,3	32,7	59,8

Table 11. The types of symptoms in study group.

Study group			
Heartburn[%]	**Frequency of symptoms [%]**		
yes/not	**Occasional**	**Once a week**	**Everyday**
62,7/37,3	35,4	15,8	11,4

Table 12. The frequency of heartburn symptoms in the study group.

UBT showed that in the study of 81 (50.9%) dyspeptic patients, were infected with *H. pylori*, and ELISA tests were positive in 79 (49.7%) of patients. HelicoTest was positive in 88 (55.3%) of patients (Fig.6).

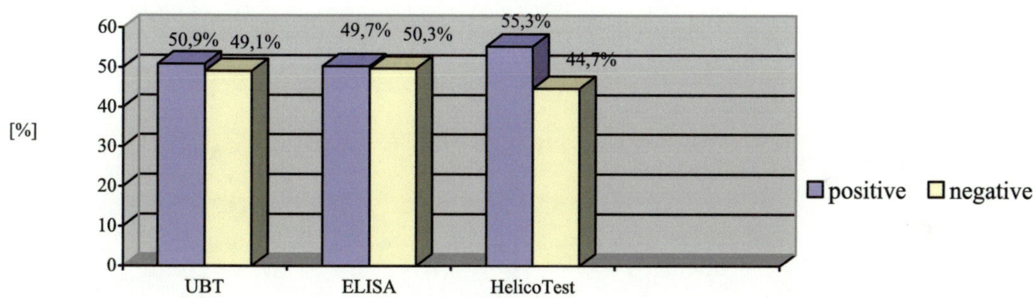

Fig. 6. The prevalence of *H. pylori* infection in the study group (p>0,05).

The increasing antibody level on ELISA showed the increasing probability of returning a positive UBT. For ELISA tests a positive result was defined as an antibody level of 1.12 (U/ml) using the Generalized Linear Model and 1.07 (U/ml) using the Generalized Additive Model. The IgG levels and the probability of *H. pylori* infection by UBT test is shown below (Fig.7).

The HelicoTest showed the highest prevalence of *H. pylori* infection, but the mean ELISA level by positive HelicoTest and negative UBT was 0.86 U/ml. The kappa coefficient for study group was 0.92 for UBT and ELISA and 0.66 for UBT and HelicoTest. The McNemary test showed no statistical differences in prevalence of *H. pylori* infection (Tab.13).

The majority of the young population tested had moderate dyspeptic symptoms. Analysis of the data showed little difference in detection of *H. pylori* among patients with acute, moderate, or mild dyspeptic symptoms, with patients with acute dyspeptic symptoms having the highest mean level of IgG (4.18 U/ml), (Fig.8).

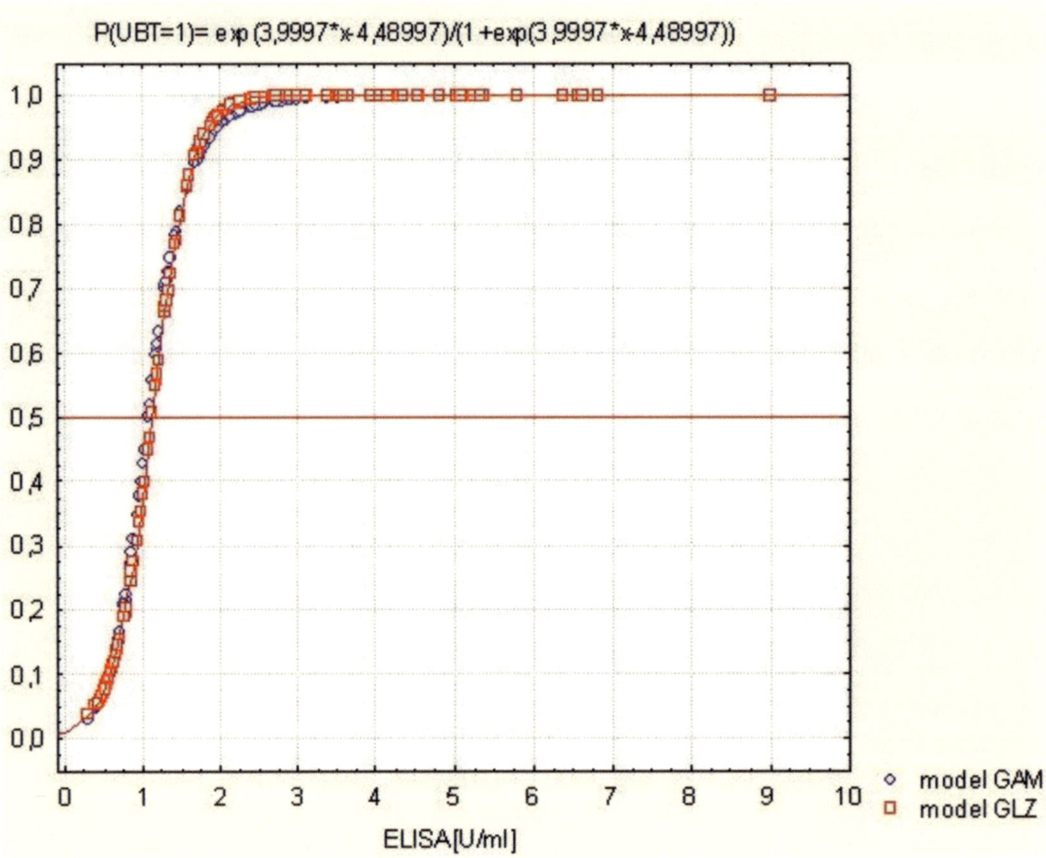

Fig. 7. The probability of *H. pylori* infection by UBT and IgG level in the study group by GAM and GLZ.

Tests	Study Group n	x^2	p
UBT test and ELISA	159	0,29	0,593
UBT test and HelicoTest	159	2,33	0,157

Table 13. Test McNemary – for study group UBT, ELISA and HelicoTEST.

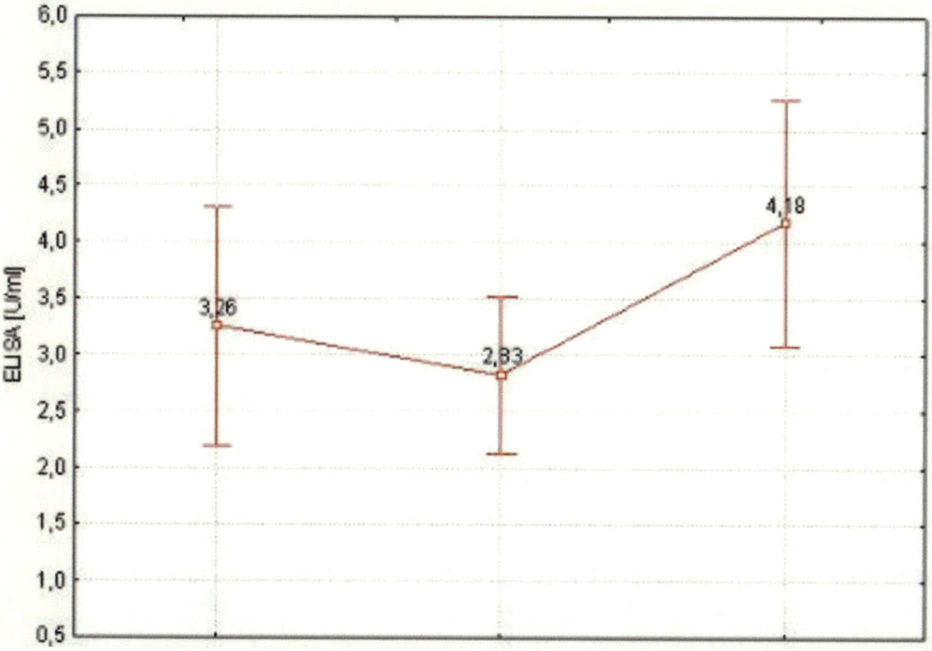

Fig. 8. The mean IgG level (U/ml) with mild, moderate and severe dyspeptic symptoms.

7. Discussion

Dyspepsia is an extremely common disorder affecting an estimated 40% of the world's population. Only a minority of patients who experience symptoms will seek medical care, but dyspepsia still accounts for 5-7% of all visits to primary care physicians. Approximately 60% of young individuals reporting symptoms have FD, with the majority of these having no underlying organic cause of their symptoms. In countries with a high prevalence of *H. pylori* infection the "test and treat strategy" is a major way to manage undiagnosed dyspepsia. The economic models suggest that in populations of low *H. pylori* prevalence managing dyspepsia with empiric acid suppression therapy is a more cost-effective method.

Noninvasive testing for *H. pylori* infection is the main mode of testing for the young dyspeptic population. The correlation between the level of *H. pylori* IgG antibodies and UBT test is largely unknown as there is little research available which examines undiagnosed dyspepsia in patients under 45 years of age in a primary care setting. *H. pylori* infection is thought to be the most common factor for morbidity and mortality in upper digestive tract diseases.

We aimed to determinate the prevalence *H. pylori* infection and dyspeptic syndrome. In the USA patients under 55, and in Canada patients under 50, along with any patients suffering from dyspepsia without alarm symptoms should be tested for *H. pylori* infection and treated appropriately to control the symptoms (6,25). The optimal age threshold for endoscopy is unclear, and it is good to not that over half of the endoscopy results will not show any organic changes in standard endoscopy.

Research on high magnifying endoscopy and chromoendoscopy has showed that new methods are superior to standard endoscopy for diagnosis of *H. pylori* gastritis and finding some mucosal and capillary structures (34).

Noninvasive *H. pylori* testing is even more important now than in the past because dyspeptic problems are increasingly seen in the primary care setting, and diagnosis of *H. pylori* infection is important to the treatment of these patients. Past studies have shown that in a population with a high prevalence of *H. pylori* infection, the "test and treat" strategy is the best option (12). Overuse NSAID's and in patients with risk factors, using cardioprotective doses of aspirin, eradication of *H. pylori* can be recommended.

The new classification of functional dyspepsia by Suzuki is based on a patient-centered approach based on the highest index of symptoms (24,28). We still do not know why the symptoms of dyspepsia fluctuate in the short-term. The strategy of rescreening *H. pylori* infection and eradication in high-risk population has already started (11,30,33).

The European Helicobacter Study Group (EHSG) was founded in 1987 to promote multidisciplinary research into the pathogenesis of *H. pylori* as a cause of upper gastrointestinal tract diseases, and how the treatment of *H. pylori* will aid in the prevention of gastric cancer (16).The EHSG has organized many annual consensus meetings and published current concepts regarding the management of *H. pylori* infection in Maastricht I, II, III and Maastricht IV (18,19,20).

The data in this study confirms that there is a correlation between the level of IgG antibodies and positive UBT test. There are some patients with dyspepsia and borderline results for *H. pylori* tests, and this is a problem that will require more research in the future (22). Right now, we strongly advise repeating the test in those patients whose symptoms persist because there is a correlation in the age and the prevalence of *H. pylori* infection in young dyspeptic patients and positive UBT test (21). There is a need to retest the population with dyspeptic symptoms and positive HelicoTest and negative UBT.

8. Conclusion

The level of IgG ELISA is a good predictor of probability of positive UBT. Serological testing by HelicoTest showed the highest prevalence *H. pylori* infection in young undiagnosed dyspeptic patients. Follow-up of these patients will be important to observe symptom relief and fluctuation in young dyspeptic patients.

9. References

[1] Agreus L, Talley N, Sheen A, et al. Predictors and non-predictors of symptom relive in dyspepsia consultations in primary care. *Digestive Diseases* 2008; 26:248-255.

[2] Aro P, Talley NJ, Agréus L, Johansson SE, Bolling-Sternevald E, Storskrubb T, Ronkainen J. Functional dyspepsia impairs quality of life in the adult population. *Aliment Pharmacol Ther.* 2011 Jun;33(11):1215-24.

[3] Barton P, Moayyedi P, Talley N, Vakil N, Delaney B. A second-order simulation model of the cost-effectiveness of managing dyspepsia in the United States. *Med Decis Making* 2008; 28: 44–55.

[4] Bolling-Sternevald E, Ronkainen P, Storskrubb T, Talley NT, Junghard O, Agreus L. Do Gastrointestinal Symptoms Fluctuate in the Short-Term Perspective? The Kalixanda Study. *Dig Dis* 2008;26:256-263.

[5] Celiński K et al. The effects of environmental factors on the prevalence of Helicobacter pylori infection in inhabitants of Lublin province. *Ann Agric Environ Med* 2006,13,185-191.

[6] Chey WD, Wong BC. American College of Gastroenterology guideline on the management of *H. pylori* infection. *Am J Gastroenterol* 2007;102:1808-25.

[7] Chiba N, Veldhuyzen Van Zanten SJ, Escobedo S, Grace E, Lee J, Sinclair P, et al. Economic evaluation of *Helicobacter pylori* eradication in the CADET-Hp randomized controlled trial of *H. pylori*-positive primary care. *Aliment Pharmacol Ther* 2004 Feb 1;19(3):349-58.

[8] Delaney B, Ford AC, Forman D, Moayyedi P, Qume M.WITHDRAWN: Initial management strategies for dyspepsia. *Cochrane Database Syst Rev.* 2009 Oct 7;(4):CD001961.

[9] Diagnosis of *Helicobacter pylori*: Invasive and non-invasive tests. C. Ricci et al. *Best Practice and Research Clinical Gastroenterology* 2007;21(2):299-313.

[10] El-Omar EM, Banerjee S, Wirz A, McColl KE. The Glasgow Dyspepsia Severity Score – a tool for the global measurement of dyspepsia. *Eur J Gastroenterol Hepatol* 1996;8(10):967-71.

[11] Fock K, Talley N, Moayyedi P, Hunt R. Asia-Pacific consensus guidelines on gastric cancer prevention. *Journal of Gastroenterology and Hepatology*. 2008;23:351-365.

[12] Ford AC, Qume M, Moayyedi P, et al. Helicobacter pylori "test and treat" or endoscopy for managing dyspepsia: an individual patient data meta-analysis.*Gastroenterology* 2005;128:1838-44.

[13] Jones R. Lydeard S: Dyspepsia in the community: A follow-up study. *Br J Clin Practi*1992;46:95-97.

[14] Kivi M, Tindberg Y. *Helicobacter pylori* occurrence and transmission: a family affair? *Scand J Infect Dis* 2006;38:407-17.12. Talley N, Ruff K, Jiang X. The Rome III Classification of Dyspepsia: Will It Help Research? *Digestive Diseases* 2008;26(3):203-209.

[15] Lane AJ, Murray LJ, Noble S, et al.: Impact of *Helicobacter pylori* eradication on dyspepsja health resource use, and quality of life in the Bristol Helicobacter project: randomised controlled trial. *BMJ* 2006; 332: 199-204.

[16] Lai L.H., Sung J.J.Y.: *Helicobacter pylori* and benign upper digestive disease. *Best Pract. Res. Clin. Gastroeterol.* 2007, 21:261-279

[17] Mahadeva S, Yadav H. et al. Ethnic variation, epidemiological factors and quality of life impairment associated with dyspepsia in urban Malaysia. *Aliment Pharmacol Ther.* 2010; 31(10):1141-51.

[18] Malfertheiner P: The Maastricht recommendations and their impact on general practice. *Eur J Gastroenterol Hepatol* 1999; suppl 2: S63-S73.

[19] Malfertheiner P, Megraud F, O'Morain C, et al. and the European *Helicobacter pylori* Study Group (EHPSG). Current concepts in the management of *Helicobacter pylori* infection – the Maastricht 2-2000 consensus report. *Aliment Pharmacol Ther* 2002; 16: 167-80.

[20] Malfertheiner P, Megraud F, O'Morain C, Bazzoli F, El-Omar E, Graham D, et al. Current concepts in the management of *Helicobacter pylori* infection: the Maastricht III consensus report. *Gut* 2007;56:772-81.
[21] Palka M, Tomasik T et al. The reliability of ELISA in predicting *H. pylori* infection in dyspeptic population under age 45. *Med Sci Monit* 2010;16(1):24-28.
[22] Sufi R, Golam M, Anisur M et al. Non-invasive diagnosis of H. pylori infection: Evaluation of serological test with and without current infection marker. World Journal of Gastroenterology 2008;14(8):1231-1236.
[23] SungLau JY, Sung JJ, Metz DC, Howden CW. Systematic review of the epidemiology of complicated peptic ulcer: incidence, recurrence, risk factors and mortality. *Gastroenterology* 2008; 134 (Suppl. 1): A32.
[24] Suzuki H, Nishihiro N, Hibi T. Therapeutic strategies for functional dyspepsia and the introduction of Rome III classification. *Journal of Gastroenterology* 2006;41(6):513-523.
[25] Talley NJ, Vakil N. Guidelines for the management of dyspepsia. *Am J Gastroenterol* 2005;100:2324-37.
[26] Thijs JC, Kleibeuker JH. The management of uninvestigated dyspepsia in primary care. *Minerva Gastroenterol Dietol* 2005;51(3):213-24.
[27] Tytgat G. Long-term GERD management: the individualized approach. *Drugs Today 2006*;42 suppl.B;23-26.
[28] Vakil V, et al. The Montreal definition and classification of gastro-esophageal reflux disease: a global evidence-based consensus. *Am.J. Gastroenterol.*2006,101:1900-1920.
[29] Van Zanten et al An evidence-based approach to the management of uninvestigated dyspepsia in era of *Helicobacter pylori. Canadian Medical Association Journal* 2000;162 (suppl 12):S3-23.
[30] Van Zanten SV, Wahlqvist P, Talley NJ, Halling K, Vakil N, Lauritsen K, Flook N, Persson T, Bolling-Sternevald E; STARS II Investigators. Randomised clinical trial: the burden of illness of uninvestigated dyspepsia before and after treatment with esomeprazole--results from the STARS II study. *Aliment Pharmacol Ther.* 2011 Oct;34(7):714-23.
[31] Wildner-Christensen M et al. Risk factors for dyspepsia in general population: NSAID, cigarette smoking and unemployment are important than *Helicobacter pylori* infection. *Scand J Gastroenterol.* 2006.41(2):149-54.
[32] Wyeth JW. Functional gastrointestinal disorders in New Zealand. *J Gastroenterol Hepatol.* 2011 Apr;26 Suppl 3:15-8.
[33] Yeh J, Karen M, Kuntz et al. Exploring the cost-effectiveness of *Helicobacter pylori* screening to prevent gastric cancer in China in anticipation of clinical trial results. *Int Journal of Cancer* 2009;124:157-166.
[34] Can Gonen et al. Comparison of high magnifying endoscopy and standard videoendoscopy for the diagnosing oh helicobacter pylori gastritis in routine clinical practice: A prospective study. Helicobacter 2009;14:(1)12-21.

2

Comparison of Detection Methods for Mycoplasmas of Significance to the Poultry Industry

R. Jarquin[1] and I. Hanning[2]
[1]*University of Arkansas, Department of Poultry Science, Fayetteville AR,*
[2]*University of Tennessee, Department of Food Science and Technology, Knoxville, USA*

1. Introduction

1.1 Description of *Mycoplasma*

Mycoplasmas sp. are prokaryote pseudo bacteria that lack a cell wall but have a cell membrane. The name *Mycoplasma* is derived from this characteristic, molli meaning "soft" and cute meaning "skin". *Mycoplasmas* are taxonomically placed in the Class Mollicutes, Order Mycoplasmatales, and Family Mycoplasmataceae. This genus is distinguished from the other genera in the family by a growth requirement for cholesterol and an inability to hydrolyze urea. Members of the genus have a small genome (580 to 1350 Kb) and relatively low G+C % content (Papaszi et al. 2003). The small genome size is clearly reflected by the reduced metabolic capabilities of *Mycoplasmas*. *Mycoplasmas* lack pathways for cell wall production and biosynthesis of purines and also lack a functional tricarboxylic acid (TCA) cycle and a cytochromemediated electron transport–chain system. These organisms must obtain many of the necessary nutrients needed to sustain the organism from the environment. For this reason, *Mycoplasmas* are obligate parasites. This characteristic is also reflected in the ideal culturing temperature (37^{0}C) the same body temperature as that of humans and many animals.

Mycoplasmas are the smallest self-replicating organisms. They were discovered in the late 1800's after being isolated from blood serum that had been enriched with cholesterol. In the 1950's Klinenberrger discovered a loss of the cell wall in the organism when she noticed that the *Mycoplasmas* were still able to divide even after being treated with antibiotics specific for inhibition of cell wall production. Currently, there are more than 120 named *Mycoplasma* species (http://www.ncbi.nlm.nih.gov/).

1.2 Mechanisms of pathogenesis

Mycoplasmas have a variety of animal hosts including humans and are capable of producing disease in many of these hosts. Of the 120 named species, 20 infect poultry with *Mycoplasma gallisepticum* and *Mycoplasma synoviae* being most commonly isolated from chickens (Kleven

2008). *Mycoplasmas* typically cause respiratory diseases in their host and in chickens the disease is characterized by coughing, nasal discharge, and air sac lesions, but in some infections no clinical symptoms appear (Feberwee et al. 2005a).

Although *Mycoplasmas* are typically isolated from the respiratory tract, they have also been isolated from the reproductive organs, brain and eyes of poultry. Once infected, *Mycoplasmas* must adhere to the surfaces of epithelial cells for successful colonization. The molecular mechanisms of pathogenesis have been investigated and along with whole genome sequencing, much of the disease process has been described (Papazisi et al., 2002; Papazisi et al., 2003).

Research into the molecular mechanisms of *M. gallisepticum* attachment and subsequent virulence has identified a specialized terminal organelle, or bleb-like structure, that serves as an attachment tip (Papazisi et al., 2002). Other potential adhesion structures include surface proteins containing highly reiterated domains. These proteins are members of large gene families, and individual members often undergo high-frequency phase variation which is thought to promote evasion of the host immune system (Dybvig and Voelker 1996).

Current theory argues that *Mycoplasmas* remain attached to the surface of epithelial cells and invasion is either not likely or does not occur significantly (King 1993). During attachment, damage to host tissues takes place releasing nutrients that can be utilized. *Mycoplasmas* primarily infect the respiratory tract causing damage to the ciliated epithelial cells lining the trachea. Ciliostasis results and mucus is not moved upwards out of the trachea which also prevents the organism from being removed.

During attachment of *Mycoplasmas* to the surface of host cells, interference with membrane receptors or altered transport mechanisms of the host cell can occur. Although no known toxins have been described, *Mycoplasmas* can produce metabolites and enzymes that are toxic to the epithelial cells. *Mycoplasmas* may also hydrolyze phospholipids utilizing phospholipases which compromises the host cell membrane. In addition, the host cell membrane is also vulnerable to peroxide and superoxide radicals (Amikan et al. 1984).

1.3 Costs for poultry production

M. gallisepticum and M. *synoviae* are the most common poultry pathogens and can impact breeder, broiler, and egg laying production. For layer operations, reductions in egg production are estimated at $140 million annually (Peebles et al. 2006). In broilers, a reduced feed conversion efficiency, depressed growth rate, and condemnation of carcasses can be economically devastating. Losses as high as $750,000 have been reported from a single outbreak of *M. gallisepticum* (Evans et al. 2005).

Economic burdens of *M. gallisepticum* and M. *synoviae* also include the cost of monitoring and detection. Culturing is a time consuming and lengthy process requiring multiple types of media and regular man hours. Serology is more rapid, but costs are also high for this method. Molecular based approaches are less costly however the initial investment in equipment can be expensive. For some producers, especially breeders, the choice may be to utilize a combination of all three for confirmation and assured detection. This approach can be quite costly, but may be worth the investment considering the cost of a loss of a breeder flock.

2. Detection methods

Antibiotics can be used to treat poultry for a *Mycoplasma* infection, but may not be fully effective at clearing the infection (Gautier-Bouchardon et al. 2002; Reinhardt et al. 2005). In most instances, it is necessary to eradicate the entire flock. Because *Mycoplasma* infection may not result in outward symptoms, a stringent biosecurity and biosurveillance practice which can facilitate early intervention strategies are necessary to control *Mycoplasma* infections. Currently, methods for detecting *Mycoplasma* infection that are typically used include culture, serology or molecular assays. Traditional culturing is not commonly utilized because the method is time consuming, the organism is slow growing, and some fastidious strains may not be detected (Dewitt 2000). Serology is much faster than culturing, but disadvantages of serology include non-specific reactions and cross-reactions between species, mis-interpretations due to recent vaccination for *Mycoplasma*, and cost are all disadvantages (Feberwee et al. 2005b). Furthermore, antibodies to *M. gallisepticum* and *M. synoviae* may not be detected until 1 to 3 weeks post-infection (Kleven 1975). The following sections will describe these three techniques for detection and give advantages and disadvantages for each method.

2.1 Culturing

As discussed in the earlier sections, culturing of *Mycoplasma* can be quite difficult due to the fastidious nature of the organism. Typically tissue samples are acquired from the respiratory tract such as the lungs, air sacs, or trachea. If whole organs such as lungs are utilized, a lavage can be performed with phosphate buffer saline (PBS). Inhibitors may be released from the host tissues during isolation if tissues are ground, but this problem can be overcome with the addition of chemicals or antibodies or by diluting the sample.

The samples are typically enriched in a broth medium with a meat-infusion base prior to plating. *M. gallisepticum* and M. *synoviae* require cholesterol and other fatty acids as a nutrient source. Supplemental antibiotics are also added to inhibit competing organisms. Frey et al. (1968) developed a culture medium that is widely used in the United States of America (USA) and other countries for isolation of *M. gallisepticum* and *M. synoviae*. Nicotinamide adenine dinucleotide (NAD) is added for the isolation of MS, but it may be omitted for the cultivation of *M. gallisepticum*. A soft agar is typically utilized (6-8%) with a neutral pH (7.4 to 7.6) and plates incubated at 37^{0}C in a moist environment.

Colonies display a fried egg shape on agar. For confirmation, commercially available antibodies specific for *Mycoplasma* with fluorescent tags can be used as well as growth tests utilizing antiserum. Preservation of cultures is similar to preservation of most bacteria. Freezing at lower temperatures will preserve the cultures for an extended period of time and adding a cryoprotecting reagent can also extend the life of the culture.

Culturing is considered the gold standard. Isolating these organisms can be very useful for further diagnostic and future epidemiological studies. Pure cultures can be characterized phenotypically and genotypically which makes culturing advantageous over serology and molecular based detection techniques. However, due to the sensitive nature of this bacterium, culturing can be labor intensive and unsuccessful. For example, Jarquin et al. (2009) compared isolation techniques and found culturing produced the greatest number of false positives when compared with serology and molecular detection techniques. The authors suggested that the time gap from sample collection to processing may have resulted in loss of cultures. In addition, the study pointed out that freezing the tissue samples may have also affected culture recovery.

2.2 Serology

Serological based assays utilized in poultry are aimed at detecting any antibodies produced by the host in response to *Mycoplasma* infection. Blood is collected from the birds and the collected sample is allowed to separate. The serum then can be used in an antibody based assay. Assays are usually in one of three formats: plate agglutination, hemagglutination inhibition (HI), or ELISA (enzyme labeled immunosorbent assay). Plate agglutination detects IgM, while HI and ELISA detect IgG.

Plate agglutination is a very simple assay in which serum is mixed with *Mycoplasma* antigens on a glass slide and positive results are can be rapidly visualized by clumping due to the antibody binding with the antigens. Plate agglutination detects IgM antibodies which are pentamers and thus, bind well to antigens. The general term agglutinin is used to describe antibodies that agglutinate to antigens. When the antigen is an erythrocyte the term hemagglutination is used. For *Mycoplasma* specifically, the plate agglutination is an assay where serum is mixed with antigens specific for *M. gallisepticum* and M. *synoviae*.

Because hemagglutination inhibition (HI) detects IgG, infection cannot be detected as early as with HI compared to plate agglutination. The assay is performed in a microtiter plate composed of 96 wells. Like plate agglutination, positive results are visualized as a cloud (inhibition of agglutination of erythrocytes) due to the antibody-antigen binding. A microtiter plate can be used where each well has a varying concentration of antibody-antigen. In this way, it is possible to quantify the amount of antibodies present in the serum sample. There are false negative results from plate agglutination and HI for two reasons: 1) early during the infection, not enough antibodies have been produced for the test to detect them (lack of sensitivity), and 2) the quality of the HI and plate agglutination antigens will impact the assay as insufficient titer of antigen will produce false negatives. These serum antigens vary considerably in titers and quality. Hence the need for internal quantitative controls is necessary to make sure each new bottle of antigen has the same or similar titer as the previous one.

Plate agglutination and HI assays are both prone to false positives. Several factors can lead to false positives but the primary contributor is vaccination with *mycoplasma* vaccines. Vaccination simulates the production of antibodies that can circulate for 2 to 5 weeks. Contaminated serum, frozen and thawed serum, and cross-reactions to other antibodies can also cause false positives. False positive reactions can be reduced by heating serum to 56°C for 30 minutes or by diluting serum (Butcher 2007). Typically, plate agglutination assays are more sensitive, but HI assays are more specific.

ELISA is the third type of antibody detecting assay. In this assay, antibodies or antigens are bound to the wells of a microtiter plate. The wells then are filled with diluted serum and given time for the binding reaction to occur. The wells are washed and a secondary antibody or antigen that is tagged with an enzyme-labeled anti-species conjugate. The addition of the enzyme chromogen reagent causes the color to develop. The amount of bound antibody or antigen is directly proportional to the intensity of the color developed. Thus, positive reactions can be visualized by noting a color change. The level of antibody present in the sample can be quantified by measuring the color intensity by spectrophotometry and extrapolating the value from a standard curve.

HI and ELISA are typically used as conformational assays for the simple plate agglutination assay. HI and ELISA are comparatively more labor intensive and thus, not utilized as a primary method. These two methods also take more time than simple plate agglutination.

2.3 Molecular

Molecular based techniques have become increasingly popular. Polymerase chain reaction (PCR) assays which target and detect specific nucleic acid sequences, can give results in less than 24 hrs. Real-time PCR also detects specific nucleic acid sequences but utilizes a fluorescent based system so the amplification of the target can be monitored during the reaction. Real-Time PCR has additional advantages over traditional PCR including: 1) real time is more rapid and can be accomplished in as little as 40 minutes; 2) no post amplification processes are required which decreases total detection time, cost in terms of materials, and hazardous waste; 3) are more sensitive - some real time assays can detect as few as 10 template copies per 5µl sample; 4) questionable results can be confirmed using melting curves.

Most PCR based methods require the sample be suspended in a non-nutrient medium. Specific to poultry, cleft palentine swabs are usually performed and the swab is then suspended in nuclease free water to release the sample from the swab. Samples are subsequently heated to boiling which lyses the cells and releases the nucleic acids. Centrifugation of this preparation collects debris in the pellet while target nucleic acids remain in the supernatant.

There are several molecular assays available for detection of *M. gallisepticum* and *M. synoviae*. Jarquin et al. (2009) and Hess (2007) utilized primers that targeted the 16S ribosomal subunit. Carli and Eygor (2003) performed detection of M. *gallisepticum* with primers that were specific for a lipoprotein gene. Hammond et al. (2009) designed their primer set to target the *vhlA* gene. The *vhlA* gene is typically utilized for genotyping and differentiating strains (Hong et al. 2004). Thus, the authors were able to detect and sequence the PCR product which facilitated epidemiological tracking efforts. Ramirez et al. (2006) targeted the interspacer region (ISR) between the 16S and 23S rRNA genes to detect and distinguish M. *synoviae* from 22 other poultry *Mycoplasmas*. Raviv et al. (2007) used the same approach for M. *gallisepticum*. All of these different primer sets have not been compared therefore it is not known whether one primer set is more accurate or sensitive than another.

3. Intervention

As discussed earlier, intervention measures are typically not performed for infected birds. A constant monitoring program is a key to early intervention. In addition, a strict biosecurity protocol is also very helpful for preventing infections with M. *gallisepticum* and M. *synoviae*. Entire flocks can become infected in 2 to 10 days (Feberwee et al. 2005a) and given that antibiotics may take 3 days to be effective, the infection can be difficult to control once it has begun. Thus, the course of action is dependent on many factors including the type of birds that are being produced. The next section will discuss three types of production operations and how *M. gallisepticum* and *M. synoviae* are controlled in these operations.

3.1 Breeders

Primary breeder operations are by far the most expensive of all three types of operations. In these system, genetic lines of birds are well established and specific traits are maintained through genetic selection. Operations typically utilize farms for production however the farms are state of the art and kept extremely clean. The cost of one bird can be as great as $5,000 and thus much time and effort is invested into maintaining a healthy population.

Primary breeders operate under the National Poultry Improvement Plan (NPIP; USDA 2009). The NPIP was formed in 1935 to target *Salmonella gallinarum* and *S. pullorum*. At this time, these bacteria were economically devastating to producers. Through cooperative vaccination and biosecurity, *S. gallinarum* and *S. pullorum* were eradicated from the U.S. Currently, *M. gallisepticum* and *M. synoviae* are a main focus of this program. Primary Breeders operating under the NPIP must comply with the program regulations that include the vending of *M. gallisepticum* and *M. synoviae* free birds.

Due to the high cost of primary breeder birds, infection with *M. gallisepticum* and *M. synoviae* are monitored frequently. Although the cost of monitoring can be expensive, given the cost of primary breeder birds, the investment in diagnostic assays is relatively low compared the potential cost of a loss of a flock. To control infection, breeders typically destroy entire flocks if *M. gallisepticum* or *M. synoviae* outbreaks occur. Since vending infected birds is not allowed under the NPIP program, eradication is the only solution.

3.2 Broilers

Many large scale broiler operations house anywhere from 15,000 to 30,000 birds per house. Each bird is given approximately 1 sq. ft. of space. Due to the proximity of the birds, infection spreads rapidly. In a controlled setting, Feberwee et al. (2005b) designed a model to measure the rate of *M. gallisepticum* transmission. In this study, all birds were housed in separate cages that were 65 cm apart (approximately 2 feet). They found transmission occurred within 14 days from infected to uninfected birds. This study primarily focused on transmission via aerosols. However, in a broiler operation there are many other factors and modes of transmission including feed and water.

For broiler operations, the course of action a producer takes is dependent on the time of infection. Broilers are typically raised for a total of 42 days prior to slaughter. Infection of young birds can lead to large losses. Younger birds have an immature immune system and cannot clear the infection. Vaccination can be done at the hatchery but vaccination is not always fully effective at preventing infection. In addition to loss of birds due to death, producers may suffer economic losses because M. *gallisepticum* and *M. synoviae* infections can reduce production parameters, and cause plant condemnations due to airsaculitis. Thus, even if the infection can be treated, a reduced bird size at the end of the rearing period can occur. If infection occurs late in the production cycle, a producer may not suffer any losses and no course of action may be required. Control of M. *gallisepticum* and M. *synoviae* in broilers has been recently reviewed (Kleven 2008).

3.3 Layers

Egg laying production systems can also be impacted by *M. gallisepticum* and *M. synoviae*. A marked reduction in egg production may result from infection with *M. gallisepticum* and *M.*

synoviae. It has been reported that *M. gallisepticum* and M. *synoviae* can cause 20-30% reduction in egg production (North 1984). Furthermore, eggs with pimpled shells are also associated with *Mycoplasma* infections (Branton et al., 1995). Since egg laying hens have relatively longer periods of production compared to broilers (80 weeks or more), once infected it is nearly impossible to eliminate the infection and therefore, production can be affected for the life of the flock.

Vaccination of laying hens is performed at 12 weeks of age and delivered in the drinking water (Usman and Diarra 2008). However, *Mycoplasma* infection can be transmitted vertically. *Myocplasma* vertical transmission can be controlled by incubating eggs at a relatively higher temperature (46^{0}C). *Mycoplasmas* cannot survive this temperature, however a reduction in hatchability may result (Usman and Diarra 2008). Thus, like other production types rigid biosecurity and a constant monitoring system can reduce the risk of *Mycoplasma* infection.

4. Conclusions and future directions

Because *Mycoplasma* can be so economically devastating, control using a monitoring system and strict biosecurity are both necessary. The NPIP program has been successful in the past with eradication of other poultry significant pathogens. Whether or not *M. gallisepticum* and *M. synoviae* can be eradicated will be a matter of time. The program targets breeder operations and therefore uses a top down approach. By controlling *M. gallisepticum* and *M. synoviae* at the breeder level, it may be more effective in preventing dissemination to the production farms. One significant source of *M. gallisepticum* and *M. synoviae* is backyard flocks. These flocks are typically small and owned for personal use. These backyard chickens are exposed to more wild animals which may be sources of *M. gallisepticum* and *M. synoviae* and biosecurity is completely absent. Thus, backyard birds can serve as a potential reservoir for the pathogens.

Current research is exploring vaccines and alternatives to antibiotics. Antibiotic alternatives include treatments such as bacteriophage and recombinant vaccines. At this point, there are no treatments or preventive therapies that are 100% effective. Therefore, prevention through biosecurity and monitoring are the only options.

5. References

Amikam, D., G. Glaser, and S. Razin. 1984. *Mycoplasmas* (Mollicutes) have a low number of rRNA genes. J. Bacteriol. 158:376–78

Branton, S.L., B.D. Lott, W.R. Maslin and E.J. Day, 1995. Fatty liver hemorrhagic syndrome observed in commercial layers fed diets containing chelated minerals. Avian Dis., 39: 631-635.

Butcher, G.D. 2007. Factors to Consider in Serologic Testing for Mycoplasma gallisepticum (M. GALLISEPTICUM) and *Mycoplasma synoviae* (M. SYNOVIAE). Available at: http://edis.ifas.ufl.edu/vm093

De Wit, J. J. Technical review, detection of infectious bronchitis virus. Avian Pathol. 29:71–93. 2000

Dybvig, K., and L.L. Voelker. MOLECULAR BIOLOGY OF MYCOPLASMAS. Annu. Rev. Microbiol. 1996. 50:25–57.1996.

Evans, J. D., S. A. Leigh, S. L. Branton, S. D. Collier, G. T. Pharr, and S. M. D. Bearson. *Mycoplasma gallisepticum*: Current and developing means to control the avian pathogen. J. Appl. Poult. Res. 14:757-763. 2005.

Feberwee, A., D. R. Mekkes, D. Klinkenberg, J.C. Vernooij, A.L. Gielkens, and J.A. Stegeman. An experimental model to quantify horizontal transmission of *Mycoplasma gallisepticum*. Avian Pathol. 34: 355-61. 2005a.

Feberwee ,A., D.R. Mekkes, J.J. de Wit, E.G. Hartman, and A. Pijpers. Comparison of culture, PCR, and different serologic tests for detection of *Mycoplasma gallisepticum* and *Mycoplasma* synoviae infections. Avian Dis. 49:260-8. 2005b.

Frey M.L., R.P. Hanson, and D.P. Anderson. A medium for the isolation of avian *Mycoplasmas*. Am. J. Vet. Res., 29, 2163–2171. 1968

Gautier-Bouchardon, A.V., A.K. Reinhardt, M. Kobisch, and I. Kempf . In vitro development of resistance to enrofloxacin, erythromycin, tylosin, tiamulin and oxytetracycline in *Mycoplasma gallisepticum, Mycoplasma iowae* and *Mycoplasma synoviae*. Vet. Microbiol. 88: 47-58. 2002.

Hessa, M., C. Neubauera, and R. Hackla. Interlaboratory comparison of ability to detect nucleic acid of *Mycoplasma gallisepticum* and *Mycoplasma synoviae* by polymerase chain reaction. Avian Pathology (April 2007) 36(2), 127133. 2007.

Hong, Y., M. García, V. Leiting, D. Bentina, L. Dufour-Zavala, G. Zavala, and S.H. Kleven. Specific Detection and Typing of *Mycoplasma synoviae* Strains in Poultry with PCR and DNA Sequence Analysis Targeting the Hemagglutinin Encoding Gene *vlhA*. Avian Diseases, 48(3):606-616. 2004.

Jarquin, R., J. Schultz, I. Hanning and S. Ricke. Development of a real-time polymerase chain reaction assay for the simultaneous detection of *Mycoplasma gallisepticum* and *Mycoplasma synoviae* under industry conditions. Avian Dis. 53:73-77.2009.

King, K.W., and K. Dybvig. Mycoplasmal cloning vectors derived from plasmid pKMK1. Plasmid 31:49–59. 1993.

Kleven, S. H. Antibody response to avian *mycoplasmas*. Am. J. Vet. Res. 36:563–565. 1975.

North, M.O. Breeder Management: *In* Commercial Chicken Production manual. The Avi. Publishing Company. Inc. Westport, Connecticut, pp: 240-243, 298-321. 1984.

Papazisi, L., T. Gorton, G. Kutish, P. Markham, G. Browning, D. Nguyen, S. Swartzell, A. Madan, G. Mahairas, and S. Geary. The complete genome sequence of the avian pathogen *Mycoplasma gallisepticum* strain Rlow. 149:2307-2316. 2003.

Peebles, E.D., E.Y. Basenko, S.L. Branton, S.K. Whitmarsh, and P.D. Gerard. Effects of s6-strain *Mycoplasma gallisepticum* inoculation at ten, twenty-two, or forty-five weeks of age on the blood characteristics of commercial egg laying hens. Poul. Sci. 85:2012-2018. 2006.

Ramırez, A., C.J. Naylor, P.P. Hammond, and J.M. Bradbury. Development and evaluation of a diagnostic PCR for *Mycoplasma synoviae* using primers located in the intergenic spacer region and the 23S rRNA gene. Vet Microbiology 118: 76–82. 2006.

Raviv, Z., S. Callison, N. Ferguson-Noel, V. Laibinis, R. Wooten, and S. H. Kleven. The *Mycoplasma gallisepticum* 16S–23S rRNA Intergenic Spacer Region Sequence as a Novel Tool for Epizootiological Studies. Avian Diseases, 51(2):555-560. 2007.

Reinhardt, A.K., A. V. Gautier-Bouchardon, M. Gicquel-Bruneau, M. Kobisch, and I. Kempf Persistence of *Mycoplasma gallisepticum* in chickens after treatment with enrofloxacin without development of resistance. Vet. Microbiol. 106:129-37. 2005.

USDA 2009. National Poultry Improvement Plan. Available at: http://www.aphis.usda.gov/animal_health/animal_dis_spec/poultry/

Usman, B.A. and S.S. Diarra. Prevalent Diseases and Mortality in Egg Type Layers: An Overview. International Journal of Poultry Science 7 (4): 304-310. 2008

Part 2

Serological Diagnosis of Viral Diseases

3

Diagnostic Methods of Viral Exanthemas in Children

Klara Martinaskova[1] and Vanda Valentova[2]
[1]*J.A. Reiman´s Faculty Hospital,*
[2]*Jessenius Faculty of Medicine of CU,*
Slovakia

1. Introduction

To diagnose a causing agent of viral infections in clinical practice we can use a number of laboratory diagnostic methods and procedures. With different pathogens we use different methods. What is important is a quality of collected biological samples, time of delivery of samples to the laboratory (one hour is the best), appropriate transport in cooling box and proper medium for virological examination. Body sites and collection methods vary according to the type of infection and viral etiology. We have to take into consideration a stage of infection, incubation period, beginning of clinical appearance and dynamic of immune response. Storage temperature of samples depends on type of biological material and used medium and of course time you need to store the sample. Each type of biological sample, such as nasopharyngeal swab tampons, cerebrospinal fluid, content of skin blisters, skin biopsies, scabs, urine samples, stool samples and blood fractions such as leukocytes, plasma or sera, requires specific way of storage and transport. We introduce a review of the most commonly used diagnostic techniques in viral infections:

1. Growth and isolation of the virus in a cell culture from a specimen taken from the patient. Most commonly used are fertilized hen's egg or laboratory animals.
2. Detection of virus-specific antibodies in the blood, IgG, IgM, IgA etc. by serological testing like ELISA, hemagglutination, complement fixation, blotting, EIA and fluorescent antibodies. Levels of immunoglobulins can show us the kinetic of infection.
3. Viral antigen detection by ELISA in tissues and fluids, or by direct or indirect immunofluorescence, or immunoperoxidase.
4. Detection of virus encoded DNA and RNA (after Rt-RNA procedure) done by polymerase chain reaction (PCR)
5. Histological examination of biopsies taken from infected tissues, or lesion typical for viral infection. Looking for viral inclusion bodies, collections of replicating virus particles either in the nucleus or cytoplasm.
6. Visualization of viruses by electron microscopy or immune electron microscopy.

2. Isolation of virus from tissue cultures

Viral disease diagnosis has relied on the isolation of viral pathogens in cell cultures. This method is often slow and requires considerable technical expertise and equipment. Cell cultures are more convenient and less expensive than eggs and lab animals. Cell cultures are suitable to be examined microscopically for evidence of viral proliferation, and, they have provided a desirable environment for the detection and identification of many human viral pathogens. Viruses reach high titres when grown within susceptible cells, and culture tubes are convenient to manipulate. Cell cultures in cell monolayer can be prepared in a variety of containers, the 16- by 125-mm glass or plastic round-bottom screw-cap tube is standard.

Clinical samples collected with a polyester swab from body sites such as skin and the genital tract, are usually contaminated with microbial flora, have to be placed in viral transport medium, which contain antibiotics, a buffered salt solution, a proteinaceous substance (such as albumin, gelatin, or serum), and a pH indicator. Stool samples or other highly contaminated samples have to be suspended and filtered through 0,45 µm membrane filters, before use. Respiratory tract samples include sputum, bronchial alveolar lavage specimens, nasopharyngeal washes, aspirates and swabs and oropharyngeal swabs have to be placed in viral transport medium. Specimens which are expected to be free of microbial contamination are collected in sterile containers and are not placed in transport medium. Preservation of the viral titre and viral infectivity until cell cultures can be inoculated is essential. Keeping the samples at 2 to 8°C or on wet ice until cell culture inoculation helps preserve viral infectivity and increases the virus recovery rate (Leland, 2007).

The transport medium tube is vortexed, the swab is discarded, the liquid medium is centrifuged, and the supernatant fluid is used to inoculate the cell cultures. Cells are cultivated in defined culture media with addition of antibiotics in sterile conditions and all handling must be done in laminar flow cabinate (boxes with laminar flow of sterile air). Usually after 24 - 48 hours of incubation at 37°C cell exhibit first cytopathic changes. These changes are best seen under the inverted microscope.

Various cell cultures are suitable for cultivation and identification of different viruses. Hundreds of cell lineages are available in international cell culture catalogues, most known is ATCC (American Type Culture Collection). Examples of well-known cell types are primary rhesus monkey kidney (RhMK) cells, primary rabbit kidney cells, human lung fibroblasts (MRC-5), human foreskin fibroblasts, human epidermoid carcinoma cells (HEp-2), human lung carcinoma cells (A549), and others (Leland, 2007).

Degenerative changes in monolayer cells provide evidence of viral presence. Viruses are quantified in suspension of infected cells, and are classified by number of viral plaques. The plaque is identified as a focus of cytopathic changes (swelling, shrinking, and rounding of cells to clustering, syncytium formation, and, in some cases, complete destruction of the monolayer), around the one infected cell.

3. Animal tissue cultures

In addition to use of cell cultures in virology, it's possible to use tissue cultures for virus isolation. Fertile hen's eggs and laboratory animals like newborn mice are very useful for the isolation of certain viruses. Brain cells of newborn mouse are convenient for replication of Coxsackie virus, for which cell cultures are not suitable. Methods for identification of replicating viruses in living organisms are same like in cell cultures, hemagglutination or immunofluorescence using print technique. Immunofluorescence can be used on tissue sections, cultured cell lines, or individual cells and is only limited to fixed (i.e., dead) cells. Direct or indirect immunofluorescence can be used for the detection of virus antigen, whereas indirect immunofluorescence is virtually always used for the detection of antibody. Cells from the culture are immobilized onto glass slide. Specific monoclonal or polyclonal sera raised against the viral antigen can be used. Monoclonal sera offer the advantage of increased sensitivity and specificity. Samples have to be blocked with specific sera, than primary and potentially secondary antibody is added and detected with fluorescent microscope. Isolation and identification of unknown virus is very difficult. For ordinary isolation our material is sent to laboratory with specific request, for example to isolate enterovirus, etc. (Rajčáni ,Čiampor, 2006).

4. Polymerase Chain Reaction (PCR)

Detection of virus encoded DNA and RNA (after Rt-RNA procedure) is done with polymerase chain reaction. The polymerase chain reaction (PCR) is a scientific technique used to amplify a single or a few copies of a piece of DNA across several orders of magnitude, generating thousands to millions of copies of a particular DNA sequence.

Almost all PCR applications use a heat-stable DNA polymerase. This DNA polymerase enzymatically assembles a new DNA strand from nucleotides, by using single-stranded DNA as a template and DNA primers, which are required for initiation of DNA synthesis.

PCR method uses thermal cycling, heating and cooling of the PCR sample to a defined series of temperature steps, necessary first to denature (physically separate) two strands in a DNA double helix at a high temperature 94°C.

Next step is the hybridization, when at a lower temperature of 50°C two complementary primers are attached to the 3´ends of separated strands of the target segment of DNA. PCR primers are usually short, chemically synthesized oligonucleotides, with a length not more than 30 (usually 18–24) nucleotides. They need to match the beginning and the end of the DNA fragment to be amplified and are then used as the template in DNA synthesis by the DNA polymerase to selectively amplify the target DNA.

Third step is a proper synthesis of the new complementary DNA strand. As a starting point for DNA synthesis are used PCR primers, because DNA polymerases, can only add new nucleotides to an existing strand of DNA.

Another type of nucleic acid detection is nucleic acid hybridization with virus-specific probes detecting specific viruses. Molecular techniques such as dot-blot, Western blot and Southern-blot depend on the use of specific DNA/RNA probes for hybridization. The specificity of the reaction depends on the conditions used for hybridization. A mixture containing the molecule to be detected is applied directly on a membrane as a dot. This is then followed by detection by either nucleotide probes. Dot blots can only confirm the presence or absence of a viral nucleic acid which can be detected by the DNA probes.

5. Serology

When the immune system of a patient encounters a virus, it produces specific antibodies which bind to the virus and mark it for destruction. The presence of these antibodies is often used to determine whether a person has been exposed to a given virus in the past. Serology is the detection of rising titres of antibodies between an acute and convalescent stage of infection, or the detection of IgM in primary infection. There are several serology techniques that can be used depending on the antibodies being studied. These include: ELISA, agglutination, precipitation, complement-fixation, fluorescent antibodies or Western blot.

In serologic diagnostic, concrete virus acts as a single antigen, although it represents wide antigen mosaic.

5.1 Agglutination reaction and virus neutralization reaction

Agglutination reaction and virus neutralization reaction measure effect of antibodies on infectivity of the virus, in determinate sera concentration (Rajčáni & Čiampor, 2006).

5.2 Agglutination test

When bacteria, antigen-coated particles, or cells in suspension are mixed with antibody directed to their surface determinants, reaction leads to agglutination of cells or particles carrying the antigen. All antibodies can theoretically agglutinate particulate antigens but IgM, due to its high valence, is particularly good.

Agglutination tests can be used in qualitative or quantitative manner, for presence of antibody or to measure the level of antibodies to particulate antigens.

Serial dilutions of a sample are made to be tested for antibody and then a fixed number of red blood cells or bacteria or other antigen is added. The maximum dilution that gives visible agglutination is called the titer.

When the antigen is an erythrocyte the term hemagglutination is used.

Hemagglutination tests can be subclassified depending on whether they detect antibodies against red cell determinants (direct and indirect hemagglutination) or against compounds artificially coupled to red cells (passive hemagglutination).

- Direct hemagglutination – red cells are agglutinated using IgM antibodies recognizing epitopes
- **Paul-Bunnell test**: diagnosis of infectious mononucleosis, detects circulating cross-reactive antibodies that combine with antigens of an animal of a different species induce the agglutination of sheep or horse erythrocytes
- Indirect hemagglutination – detects IgG antibodies that react with antigens present in the erythrocytes but which by them cannot induce agglutination. A second antibody directed to human immunoglobulins is used to induce agglutination.
- **Coombs test**: used to test for autoimmune hemolytic anemia.
- Passive hemagglutination - it is possible to coat erythrocytes with a soluble antigen (e.g. viral antigen, a polysaccharide or a hapten) and use the coated red blood cells in an agglutination test for antibody to the soluble antigen

5.3 Complement fixation reaction

Complement fixation reaction can be used to detect the presence of either specific antibody or specific antigen in a patient's serum. The complement system is a system of serum proteins that react with antigen-antibody complexes resulting in the formation of membrane pores and therefore destruction of the cell. If the patient's serum contains antibodies against the concrete virus, they will bind to the antigen to form antigen-antibody complexes. The complement proteins will react with these complexes and be depleted. When commonly used sheep red blood cells with their own antibody complexes are added, there will be no complement left in the serum. If no antibodies against the concrete virus are present, the complement will not be depleted and it will react with the sheep red blood cells antibody complexes, lysing the red blood.

5.4 Enzyme-Linked Immunosorbent Assay (ELISA)

Enzyme-linked immunosorbent assay (ELISA) serves for detection and quantification of specific antibodies in sera. A liquid sample is added onto a solid phase with special binding properties and is followed by adding antibodies and other reagents, incubated and washed. The result is a color development by the product of an enzymatic reaction. The quantity of the analyte is measured by quantitative detection of intensity of transmitted light by spectrophotometric method.

A wide variety of assay principles can be used in ELISA techniques.

In competitive methods one component of the immune reaction is insolubilized and the other one labelled with an enzyme. The anti viral antibodies can then be quantified by their ability to prevent the formation of the complex between the insolublized and the labelled reagent.

Sandwich method is the method in which antigen is used in an insolubilized form to bind the viral antibody, which is subsequently determined by addition of labelled second antibody against the same class of antibody as the analyte antibody.

5.5 Radioimmunoassay (RIA)

Radioimmunoassay (RIA) instead of measuring color changes, radioactive substances is used to visualize viral antigens. RIA technique is very sensitive and specific, but it requires specialized equipment and special precautions and licensing, since radioactive substances are used.

For serologic examination two blood samples (5-10 ml) are needed to confirm existence of specific antiviral antibodies. First sample must be taken in the shortest possible time after clinical manifestation of viral infection, the latest 5th -6th day. In this sample, levels of antibodies are low, but specific IgM antibodies are present. Second sample should be taken after appropriate interval depending on the type of infection. In general the most convenient is convalescence time, around 21 days after clinical manifestation (Rajčáni & Čiampor, 2006), on the other hand according to Sterling (2004) the best time for second blood sample is 10 - 14 days after first blood sample examination, when first antiviral antibodies start to be detectable.

The best way is to examine both samples at once to compare titres of antibodies. It is valuable also individual serological testing, in cases of high antiviral antibody titres.

Very important is to interpret the results in right way, by specialist. In case of immunodeficient or immunosupressed patients results are not valuable (Sterling, 2004).

5.6 Fluorescent antibodies or immunofluorescence

Fluorescent antibodies or immunofluorescence is used primarily on biological samples. Technique uses the specificity of antibodies to their antigen to target fluorescent dyes within a cell, and therefore allows visualization of the distribution of the target molecule through the sample. Immunofluorescence can be used on tissue sections, cultured cell lines, or individual cells. In virus diagnosis, we can use specific antibodies to concrete viral capsid proteins or to their nucleic acid specific sequences.

Primary, or direct, immunofluorescence uses a single antibody that is chemically linked to a fluorophore. The antibody recognizes the target molecule and binds to it, and the fluorophore it carries can be detected via microscopy.

Secondary, or indirect, immunofluorescence uses two antibodies; the unlabeled primary antibody specifically binds the target molecule, and the secondary antibody, which carries the fluorophore, recognizes the primary antibody and binds to it. Multiple secondary antibodies can bind a single primary antibody. This provides signal amplification by increasing the number of fluorophore molecules per antigen.

6. Diagnosis of hand, foot and mouth disease

Hand, foot and mouth disease is a human syndrome caused by intestinal viruses of the Picornaviridae family. The most common strains causing hand, foot and mouth disease (HFMD) are Coxsackie A virus, and Enterovirus 71.

Biological material from infected individuals must be cultivated in tissue cultures, same as used for common virus cultivation. Samples are inoculated mainly on *Macacus rhesus* or *cynomolgus* kidney tissue, or on human embryonic kidney cells, or WI 38 cells (Chonmaitree et al., 1981). Cytopathic effect on cell cultures is monitored and identified using direct immunofluorescence, PCR, or RT-PCR (Ooi et al., 2003).

Using mentioned methods it is possible to identify viral genome directly in samples from infected tissues, or in biologic samples from infected persons. Biopsies from infected patient can be examined also immunohistochemicaly to prove viral antigens, or with direct and indirect immunofluorescence.

Molecular biology methods do not serve only for verification of the virus in the samples, but also for more accurate genotypization of viruses that cause infection (Shimizu et al., 2004).

Except these diagnostic methods to identify virus causing HFMD, serologic screening can be used in clinical practice. From serologic methods, mainly ELISA is used to prove existence of virus neutralization antibodies class IgG, IgA, IgM, and anti-gangliozide antibodies GM1, GA1, GDa, GDb and GQ1b. Other standard biochemical methods can be used too.

7. Diagnosis of parvovirus B I9 infection

Diagnosis of Parvovirus B 19 infection in immunocompetent patients is primarily confirmed by detection of anti-viral antibodies. Other assays based on antigen detection have been developed, including a receptor mediated hemagglutination assay (RHA), based on interaction of Parvovirus B 19 and P antigen on human erythrocytes. Because human parvovirus B19 is unable to replicate in culture systems, viral antigens were initially obtained from acutely infected patients. Recently, human Parvovirus B 19 antigens have been expressed in different systems. However, bacterial systems for the viral antigens undergo denaturation. This phenomenon may be responsible for false negative results due to the absence of conformational epitopes. According to several authors these conformational epitopes are essential for accurate serologic diagnosis (Manaresi, 2001). In 1982 Anderson et al., developed a radioimmunoassay (RIA) for detection of specific anti - Parvovirus B 19 IgM antibodies. Later, an enzyme - linked immunosorbent assay (ELISA) was developed for the detection of specific anti-Parvovirus IgM antibodies (Anderson, 1986). This assay used virus obtained from viremic patients as an antigen source.

Specific IgM antibodies are detectable in more than 90% of cases at the end of the first week of illness and the titer and positivity rate decreased after 1 month. The sensitivity and specificity of ELISA was confirmed by Schwarz et al. (Schwarz 1988) who found that anti - Parvovirus B19 IgM could be detected for up to 20 weeks post-viremia and non-specific reactions with rheumatoid factor or Rubella were not found. Using immunoblotting, some authors also observed that the immune response after acute infection was directed initially against virus protein 2 (VP2) and secondly against virus protein (VP1) (Schwarz, 1988). IgM response against VP1 linear epitopes is more prevalent and persistent than the one directed against the VP2 linear antigen (Palmer, 1996). When the IgM response declines, an IgG immune-response against structural proteins VP1 and VP2 becomes prominent and can be detected by IFA, Western blot and ELISA. Similarly to the IgM response, specific IgG antibodies are produced against both denaturated and undenaturated VP1 and VP2 epitopes.

Parvovirus B 19 infections are responsible for variety of disorders in humans. The clinical presentation is different accordingly to the period of life at which the infection or reactivation of the virus occurs. The virus has been extensively studied as causative agent of autoimmune diseases (Peterlana, 2006).

PCR and real time-PCR improve the sensitivity of detection of viral infection and many clinical laboratories complement serologic diagnosis with PCR. However, this molecular procedure may be necessary only in particular clinical setting because anti-Parvovirus B 19 VP2 IgM has been reported to correlate with Parvovirus B 19 DNA level (Beersma, 2005). Therefore the use of PCR procedure does not add any further information to a positive serologic test.

8. Detection of concomitant virus infections

New opinions in infections, the vaccinations and associated changes of viral antigenic qualities, influence clinical symptomatology. These changes in viral factors, including virulence and tropism are possible. Co-infection with a second virus has been suggested and this theory is supported by concomitant isolation of subgenus B adenovirus with an enterovirus from three persons who died during hand, foot and mouth disease (HMFD) outbreak in Sarawak (Cardosa, 1999). Among the Singaporean patients with HEV71 infection, three had second virus isolated concurrently. However, the presence of dual viruses did not result in severe disease, although a child with HEV71 (Human enterovirus 71) and CAV16 (Coxsackie A 16) co-infection died in Singapore in 1997. An epidemic outbreak of HFMD occurred in Singapore between September and November 2000. During the epidemic, there were four HFMD-related deaths and after the epidemic, another three HFMD-related deaths. Enterovirus 71 positive fatal (n = 4) cases and non fatal controls (n = 63) were also compared. Of the 131 non fatal cases three had concomitant infections with virus bronchiolitis, right-side pneumonia (respiratory syncytial virus bronchiolitis, right-sided pneumonia, Haemophilus influenza type B meningitis), 2 had aseptic meningitis and 1 had transient drowsiness (Chong, 2003). Since June 2006 till September 2009 in Europe -in eastern region of Slovakia 295 children have been examined because of unknown exanthemas. According to complete history, physical examination, and specific viral and serological examinations, viral exanthemas were detected. Parvovirus B 19 infections were positive in 45 children, Coxsackie B3, B4, B6 serotypes of hand, foot and mouth / (HFMD) present in 25 persons. Concomitant dual infection occurred in 20 children. *Mycoplasma pneumonia* and Parvovirus B19 were the most frequent. Authors suggested that differences in clinical features of exanthemas, duration of diseases and severe diseases were a result of co-infections (Martinaskova, 2010).

9. References

Anderson, L.J.; Tsou, C., Parker, R.A. et al. Detecttion of antibodies and antigens of human parvovirus B19 by enzyme linked immunosorbent assay. J.Clinic Microbiol 1986; 24,522-526

Anderson MJ, Davis LR, Jones SE, Pattuson JR The development and use of an antibody capture radioimmunoassay for specific IgM to a human parvovirus like agent. J.Hyg.Camb 1982, 88, 309-324

Chong CY ,Chan K-P, Shah V A, WYM Ng. Lau G et al. Hand ,foot and mouth disease in Singapore a comparison fatal and non-fatal cases. Acta Pediatr. 2003; 1163-1169

Chonmaitree T, Menegus MA, Schervis-Swierkosz EM, Schwalentocker E Enterovirus 71 infection: Report of an outbreak with two cases of paralysis and review of literature. Pediatrics 1981; 67,489-493

Leland DS, Ginocchio CC Role of cell culture for virus detection in the age of technology. Clin.Microbiol.Rev.2007; 20(1): 49-78

Manaresi E, Zuffi E, Gallinella G,gentoloni G, Zerbinin ML, Musiani M Differential IgM response to conformational and linear epitopes of parvovirus B19VP1and VP2 structural proteins. J.Med.Virol 2001; 64, 67-73

Martinásková K, Koval' J Concomitant viral exanthemas in children-diagnostic challenge(Abstract) Eu J Pediatr. Dermatol. 2010 (Abstract Book 1): 52

Ooi MH, Wong SCH, Clear D, Pereira D, Krishnan S, Preston T, Tio PH,Wilson HJ, Tedman B,Kneen R, Cardosa MJ, Solomon T Adenovirus type 21-associated acute flaccid paralysis during an outbreak of hand-foot-mouth disease in Sarawak, Malaysia. Clin.Infect Dis.2003; 550-559

Palmer P, Pallier C,Leruez –Ville ,Deplanche M, Morinet Antibody response to human parvovirus B19 in patients with primary infections by immunoblot assay with recombinant with. Clin Diagn Lab Immunol. 1996; 3, 236-238

Peterlana D, Puccettu A, Corrocher R, Lunardi C Serologic and molecular detection of human Parvovirus B 19 infection. Clinica Chimica Acta 2006; 11, 161-163

Rajčáni J, Čiampor F Lekárska virológia. 2006; VEDA, Bratislava, 573p.

Schimizu H, Utama A, Onnimala N, Li Ch, Li-Bi Z, Yu-Jie M, Ponsuwanna Y, Miyamura T Molecular epidemiology of enterovirus 71 infection in the Western pacific region. Pediatrics International 2004; 46, 231-235

Sterling JC Virus infections.25. 1-25.83, In: Burns T, Breathnach. S, Cox N, Griffiths CH.Rook´s Textbook of Dermatology.7th Ed,.Victoria-Australia, Blackwell Science, 2004; 78.1.s

4

Serodiagnosis of *Peste des Petits Ruminants* Virus

Muhammad Munir[1,2], Muhammad Abubakar[3], Siamak Zohari[1,2,4] and Mikael Berg[1,2]
[1]Department of Biomedical Sciences and Veterinary Public Health, Division of Virology, Swedish University of Agricultural Sciences (SLU), Uppsala,
[2]Joint Research and Development Unit for Virology of SVA and SLU, Uppsala,
[3]National Veterinary Laboratory (NVL), Park Road, Islamabad,
[4]Immunobiology, Parasitology of the National Veterinary Institute (SVA), Uppsala,
[1,2,4]Sweden,
[3]Pakistan

1. Introduction

The Peste des Petits Ruminants (PPR) is one of the epizootic diseases of small ruminants, which is highly infectious and causes high mortality (Kitching, 1988). The clinical outcomes of the disease give it all the hallmarks of an economic and social disaster, especially in the small industries in developing nations. Given the impact on animal health and the economic relevance, PPR is regarded as an Office International des Epizooties (OIE) list A (A050) disease. The OIE and FAO are keen to control and subsequently eradicate PPR from the globe, as has been practiced for Rinderpest (RP). The first step in the eradication of a disease is accurate and reliable diagnosis. It is impossible to ascertain the magnitude and variability of a disease within susceptible populations without efficient diagnosis, which may lead to failure of the eradication program (Banyard *et al.*, 2010). In this chapter, we will review the background of PPRV research focusing on its contribution to basic virology and technological development. We will also highlight some old discoveries and will provide crucial momentum to the development of the current concepts and technologies in the serodiagnosis of this deadly disease.

1.1 An overview of *Peste des Petits Ruminants*

The PPR, a contagious viral infection of both wild and domestic cloven-hoofed small ruminants, is characterized by fever, pneumonia, profuse diarrhoea, and inflammation of the mucous membrane of the respiratory and digestive tracts (Ismail & House, 1990). Although all wild ruminants are susceptible to infection, PPR has only been diagnosed in

Gazellinae (Dorcas gazelle), Caprinae (Nubian ibex and Laristan sheep), Hippotraginae (gemsbok) and *Capra aegagrus blythi* (Sindh Ibex) (Abubakar *et al.*, 2011; Furley *et al.*, 1987).

In contrast to rinderpest (RP), which is one the best-known diseases historically, PPR was identified not long ago. The PPR virus was first detected in 1942 when Gargadennec and Lalanne realized that a RP like disease caused symptoms in sheep and goats but was not transmittable to cattle (Gargadennec & Lalanne, 1942). After demonstration in 1956 that PPRV is antigenically distinct from RP and its isolation in cell culture in 1962, Gibbs and coworkers categorized PPRV as another member of genus *Morbilliviruses* (Gibbs *et al.*, 1979). Initially, susceptible populations of sheep and goats were immunized using already available live attenuated RP vaccine, due to antigenic similarity of PPRV with the RP virus. Later, in 1989, a live attenuated PPRV vaccine was applied for disease control after its first successful attenuation [reviewed in (Sen *et al.*, 2010)]. Currently, comparison of various characteristics between PPR and RP, and rescuing the chimeric viruses for differentiation of infected and vaccinated animals (DIVA) and full genome sequencing of PPRV, have made substantial advances in understanding of the disease.

Phylogenetically, based on the fusion (F) and nucleocapsid (N) genes, PPRV can be classified into four distinct lineages (Figure 1) (Shaila *et al.*, 1996). PPRV belonging to lineages I and II are exclusively isolated from the countries of PPRV origin in West Africa. Lineage III is restricted to Middle East (Yemen, Qatar and Oman) and East Africa, although some of the viruses that belong to lineage III have also been isolated from southern India. Lineage IV is considered a new lineage comprising newly emerging viruses, and is most prevalent in Asian countries (Munir *et al.*, 2011; Shaila *et al.*, 1996). The proper understanding of lineage distribution in a specified region is essential when choosing the appropriate homologous prototype to ensure efficient immunization. The continued application of heterologous vaccine candidates hitherto not prevalent may lead to generation of novel lineages, or allow the existing population to evade protection, especially in RNA viruses. Therefore, identification of the lineage is a pre-requisite for fruitful diagnosis, epidemiology and control.

1.2 *Peste des Petits Ruminants* virus

PPR virus belong to the family *Paramyxoviridae*, order *Mononegavirales* and is a member of the genus *Morbillivirus* along with the rinderpest, canine distemper and measles viruses (Gibbs *et al.*, 1979). PPR viruses are pleomorphic in shape and are enveloped. The genome is single stranded RNA, and is enclosed in a ribonucleoprotein core together with nucleocapsid protein (Figure 2 A, B). The genome is composed of 15,948 nucleotides, which is the longest of all the *Morbillivirus* members (Bailey *et al.*, 2005). The PPRV genome encodes six genes, each responsible for transcription of a single protein in the order N, phosphoprotein (P), matrix (M), F, hemagglutinin (H) and the large RNA polymerase (L) (Figure 2, C). The P gene encodes for two additional non-structural proteins, C and V. The three viral proteins (M, F and H) are associated with the host-derived envelope. The matrix (M) protein is linked to the nucleocapsid and surface proteins (F and H) (Mahapatra *et al.*, 2006). The L protein acts as RNA dependent RNA polymerase. The association of P protein to N and L is linked to viral cycle control, transcription and translation regulation.

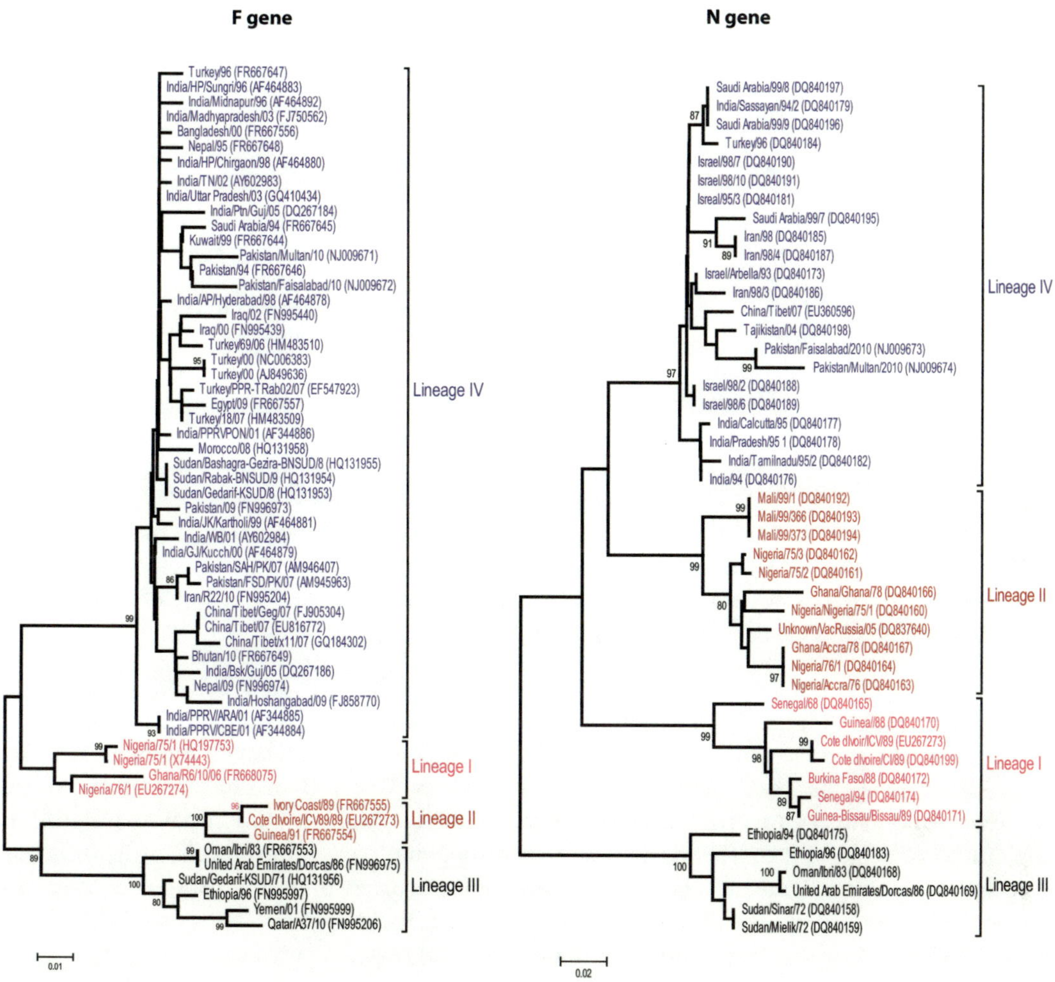

Fig. 1. Phylogenetic analysis of the F gene (left panel) and N gene (right panel) of representative PPRV isolates. Trees were generated by the neighbor-joining method in the MEGA 5.0 program. Numbers above the branches indicate neighbor-joining bootstrap values (values above 80% are shown).

2. Host response to PPRV and potential for serodiagnosis

The protective immune response is usually elicited against the surface F and H proteins of PPRV. However, among the viral proteins most of the neutralizing antibodies are directed against the H protein during PPRV infection (Diallo *et al.*, 2007). In all members of the genus *Morbillivirus* including PPRV, the N protein is the most abundant viral protein due to its presence at the extreme 3′-end of the viral genome. Owing to its high quantity during infection, the N protein is considered the most immunogenic, but the immunity produced against N protein does not protect the animals from the disease. By virtue of the nature of the H and N proteins, these remain the most acceptable targets for the design of PPRV diagnostic tools (Munir, 2011).

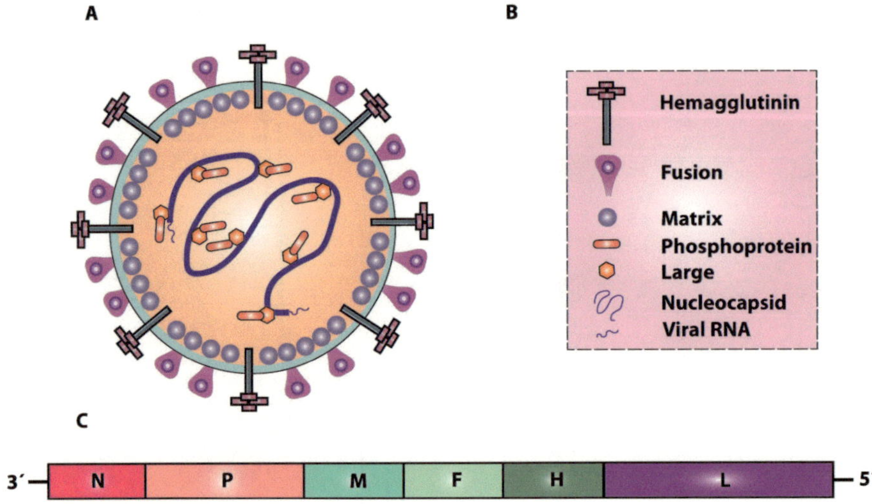

Fig. 2. A schematic illustration of the PPR virus structure. The arrangement of the viral proteins is shown in the structure (A). The names of the viral proteins present in the virus structure are shown in the box (B). The viral genome organization and arrangement of the different viral proteins in the genome are shown (C).

Based on putative amino acid sequences, hypothetically the N protein can be divided into four regions (I-IV) (Figure 3 A). Region I includes amino acids 1-120, region II includes 121-145, region III comprises amino acids 146-398, and region IV finishes with amino acids 421-525. Recently, it has been demonstrated that regions I and II are comparatively more immunogenic than regions III and IV (Choi *et al.*, 2005b). Another study demonstrated that the amino acids from 452-472 are the most immunogenic part within the N protein. It has further been summarized that there is development of earlier immune response to region I and II than region III and IV (Bodjo *et al.*, 2007). Most of the diagnostic assays for PPRV have been developed based on monoclonal antibodies (mAb) raised against the N protein (Libeau *et al.*, 1995).

The H protein of PPRV, on the other hand, is the most diverse among all the members of *Morbilliviruses*. This can be seen from the fact that the two most similar member of the genus share only 50% similarity in their H proteins. The most variable nature of H protein probably reflects the role of this protein is species specificity. If this is the case, H proteins of RP and PPR virus may have significant potential for differentiation of infected from vaccinated animals (DIVA) strategies. Since the H protein determines the cell tropism, most of the protective host immune response is raised against the H protein (Renukaradhya *et al.*, 2002). For this reason, and the preponderance of the neutralizing antibodies again the H protein, it has remained under continuous immunological pressure. The H protein is not only involved in cell-tropism but studies indicate that it may have a role as a neuraminidase. PPRV is unique among *Morbilliviruses*, which carry this function. Mapping of the functional domain, using monoclonal antibodies, has demonstrated that two regions, one at amino acids 263-368 and other at 539-609, are the most immuno-dominant epitopes (Seth & Shaila, 2001) (Figure 3 B). There is an increasing tendency to design DIVA strategies targeting the H protein of PPRV.

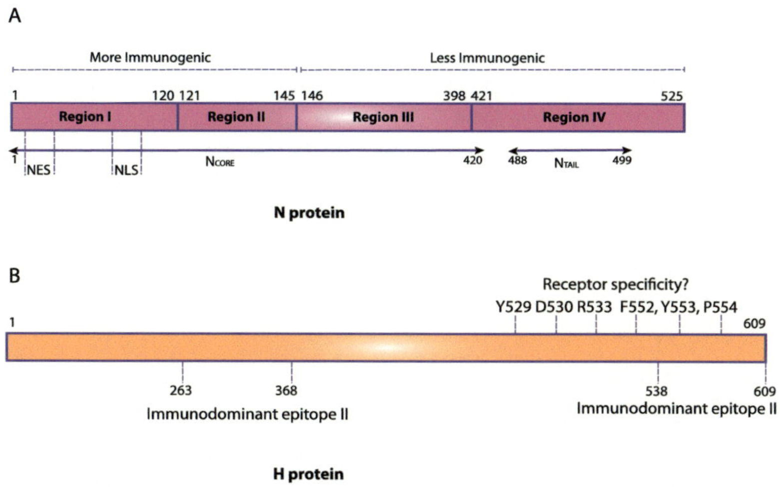

Fig. 3. Schematic illustration of the structural arrangement of the N and H proteins. The N protein is divided into four regions (I, II, III, IV) or two domains (Ncore and Ntail). The first two regions are reported to be more immunogenic than the other two. The nuclear localization and nuclear export signals are located in region I (A). Residues 263-368 and 538-609 in the H protein are considered to be immunodominant epitopes. Several amino acids in and around the second immunodominant epitope are identical to the receptor binding site for SLAM recognized for measles virus (B).

3. Specimen collection, processing and shipment

Efficient documentation and processing is the key to successful laboratory diagnosis of any pathogen. Therefore, most care must be taken to address these elements.

3.1 Documenting sample collection

Before collecting or sending any sample from animals with suspected PPR disease, the appropriate authorities should be contacted. Samples should be sent only under secure conditions and to authorized laboratories, to prevent the spread of the disease.

In the animals that survive the disease, swabs are taken from the conjunctival discharges and the nasal and buccal mucosae, and debris from oral lesions should be collected; a spatula can be rubbed across the gum and inside the lips to collect samples from oral lesions. During the very early phase of the disease, whole blood is also collected in anticoagulant for virus isolation, polymerase chain reaction (PCR) and haematology. At necropsy, lymph nodes, especially the mesenteric and bronchial nodes, lungs, spleen and intestinal mucosae should also be collected aseptically, chilled on ice and transported under refrigeration. Fragments of organs collected for histopathology are placed in 10% formalin.

3.2 Serological samples for antibody detection

At the end of the outbreak, blood can be collected for serological diagnosis. Depending upon the distance from the diagnostic laboratory and the time required for shipment, choose the best source for maintaining cold such as ice, ice pads, ice cooler or dry ice. In either case:

1. Place the glass tubes containing serum samples into mailing canisters, and put these into sealable plastic bags and seal them.
2. Every shipping icebox should contain a plastic liner. Place all the contents, such as dry ice and samples, inside this box liner.
3. Place the sealed plastic bag with canister in the dry ice box.
4. An adequate amount of dry ice is essential. Calculate according to the need as 3-4 kg of dry ice/day of shipment or 8 kg for overnight shipment. Label this amount on the box.
5. Label these boxes with the clinical specimens, not the biological specimen, and include the forms recommended by the concerned lab.
6. Inform the lab about this shipment and instruct to store these samples at -20°C.

3.3 Samples for virus isolation

Even when diagnosis has been carried out by rapid techniques, the virus should always be isolated from field samples in tissue cultures for further confirmation and research studies. Whole blood (in EDTA) should be taken for virus isolation. Samples for virus isolation should be collected during the acute stage of the disease, when clinical signs are present, and these samples should be taken from animals with high fever and before the onset of diarrhea.

3.4 Samples for antigen detection

At necropsy, samples can be collected from lymph nodes (particularly the mesenteric and mediastinal nodes), lungs, spleen, tonsils and affected sections of the intestinal tract (e.g. ileum and large intestine). These samples should be taken from euthanized or freshly dead animals. Samples for virus isolation should be transported chilled on ice. Similar samples should be collected in formalin for histopathology. Whenever possible, paired sera should be taken rather than single samples. However, in countries that are PPR-free, a single serum sample (taken at least a week after the onset of clinical signs) may be diagnostic.

4. Laboratory diagnosis of PPR

Successful implementation of control measures for PPR requires rapid, specific and sensitive methods for diagnosis. Small ruminants infected with PPR are routinely diagnosed on the basis of clinical examination, gross pathology, histological findings and laboratory confirmation (Bruning-Richardson *et al.*, 2011; Atta-ur-Rahman *et al.*, 2004). A number of serological and molecular diagnostic tests are used for the detection of PPR virus.

Conventional techniques used for PPRV detection are: agar gel immunodiffusion (AGID) (Munir *et al.*, 2009b), counter immunoelectrophoresis (CIEP) (Diallo *et al.*, 1995; Obi & Ojeh, 1989), dot enzyme immunoassay (Perl *et al.*, 1995; Obi & Patrick, 1984), differential immuno-histochemical staining of tissue sections (Saliki *et al.*, 1994), haemagglutination (HA) and haemagglutination inhibition (HI) tests (Raj *et al.*, 2008; Saravanan *et al.*, 2006; Manoharan, 2005), virus isolation (Manoharan, 2005; Brindha *et al.*, 2001), competitive enzyme-linked immunosorbent assay (c-ELISA) (Ezeibe *et al.*, 2008; Anderson *et al.*, 1991), novel sandwich ELISA (Munir *et al.*, 2009b; Anderson & McKay, 1994), immuno-capture enzyme-linked immunosorbent assay (IC-ELISA) (Abubakar *et al.*, 2008; Saravanan *et al.*, 2008; Khan *et al.*, 2007; Singh *et al.*, 2004; Libeau *et al.*, 1994), immunofiltration (Diop *et al.*, 2005), and latex agglutination tests (Keerti *et al.*, 2009).

Conventional techniques such as AGID cannot be used for routine diagnosis, as these are less sensitive and not reliable (Keerti *et al.*, 2009; Osman *et al.*, 2008). However, HA and HI tests, being simple, cheaper and comparatively sensitive, can be used for routine screening purposes in control programmes (Munir *et al.*, 2009b; Osman *et al.*, 2008). For quick diagnosis and control measures, pen-side tests such as chromatographic strip test (Aslam *et al.*, 2009; Hussain *et al.*, 2003), dot ELISA etc. that can be performed without the need for equipment or technical expertise, are highly desirable (Hussain *et al.*, 2003).

Virus isolation in cell culture can be attempted using several different cell lines. Although Vero (African green monkey) cells have been the choice for isolation and propagation of PPRV, it is reported that B95a, an adherent cell line derived from Epstein-Barr virus-transformed marmoset B-lymphoblastoid cells, is more sensitive and supports better growth of PPRV lineage IV as compared to Vero cells (Bruning-Richardson *et al.*, 2011). Techniques for virus isolation cannot be used as routine diagnostic tests as they are time-consuming and cumbersome (OIE, 2008).

Serological tests include virus neutralization and competitive ELISA assays. Both tests can distinguish peste des petits ruminants from rinderpest; this is not always possibly with older serological tests such as complement fixation. ELISAs using monoclonal antibodies have been used for serological diagnosis and antigen detection for diagnostic and screening purposes. For PPR antibody detection, competitive ELISA is a better choice as it is sensitive, specific, reliable, and has a high diagnostic specificity (99.8%) and sensitivity (90.5%) (Sreenivasa *et al.*, 2006; Choi *et al.*, 2005b; Brindha *et al.*, 2001). Immunocapture ELISA is a rapid, sensitive and virus specific test for PPRV antigen detection, and it can differentiate between RP and PPR viruses. Moreover, it is more sensitive than AGID (Abraham & Berhan, 2001).

5. Serodiagnosis of PPRV

5.1 Serum neutralization tests

This test requires the following: cell suspensions at 600,000/ml; 96-well cell culture plates; sera to be titrated (inactivated by heating to 56°C for 30 minutes); complete cell culture medium; PPRV diluted to give 1000, 100, 10 and 1 TCID50/ml. Dilute the sera at 1/5, then make a twofold dilution in cell culture medium. Mix 100 µl of virus at 1000 TCID50/ml (to give 100 TCID50 in each well) and 100 µl of a given dilution of serum (using six wells per dilution) in the wells of the cell culture plate. Arrange a series of control wells for virus and uninfected cells as follows: six wells with 100 TCID50 (100 µl) per well; six wells with 10 TCID50 (100 µl) per well; six wells with 1 TCID50 (100 µl) per well; six wells with 0.1 TCID50 (100 µl) per well; and six wells with 200 µl of virus-free culture (control cells) per well. Make the wells containing the virus controls up to 100 µl with complete culture medium, and incubate the plates for 1 hour at 37°C. Add 50 µl of cell suspension to each well. Incubate the plates at 37°C in the presence of CO_2. Read the plates after 1 and 2 weeks of incubation. The results should be as follows: 100% CPE in virus control wells of 100 and 10 TCID50, 50% CPE for the 1 TCID50 dilution, no CPE for the 0.1 TCID50 dilution, no CPE in wells where the virus had been neutralised by serum during the test, and CPE in wells where the virus had not been neutralised by serum during the test (OIE, 2008).

5.2 Haemagglutination tests

The haemagglutination test (HA) is a straightforward and rapid tool for the serological and confirmatory demonstration of antibodies against PPRV (Munir, 2011). It has been demonstrated that PPRV and MV are unique among morbilliviruses in carrying haemgglutination abilities (Wosu, 1985). The two domains within the H protein of PPRV have been demonstrated to act as immune dominant epitopes. It is now well accepted that the H protein of PPRV is not only responsible for viral attachment to cells and agglutinating erythrocytes but also cleaves sialic acid residues to help budding out the virus. Using this haemagglutinating character of PPRV, HA and HAI tests have successfully been employed for the confirmatory diagnosis of PPRV.

5.3 Haemagglutination inhibition test

This test is widely used for the quantitative measurement of PPRV antibodies usually in a suspension. In this regard, a two fold serial dilution of serum is practiced in a microwell plate. The dilution of antibodies still able to inhibit agglutination is regarded as the titer of the serum sample in the suspension. However, it is also possible to titrate the PPRV antigen using HA and HAI tests (Osman *et al.*, 2008).

5.4 Competitive ELISA

Competitive ELISA (cELISA) is one of the most extensively used tests for serological screening and diagnosis of PPRV infected animals. The detailed procedure is described below and outlined in Figure 4.

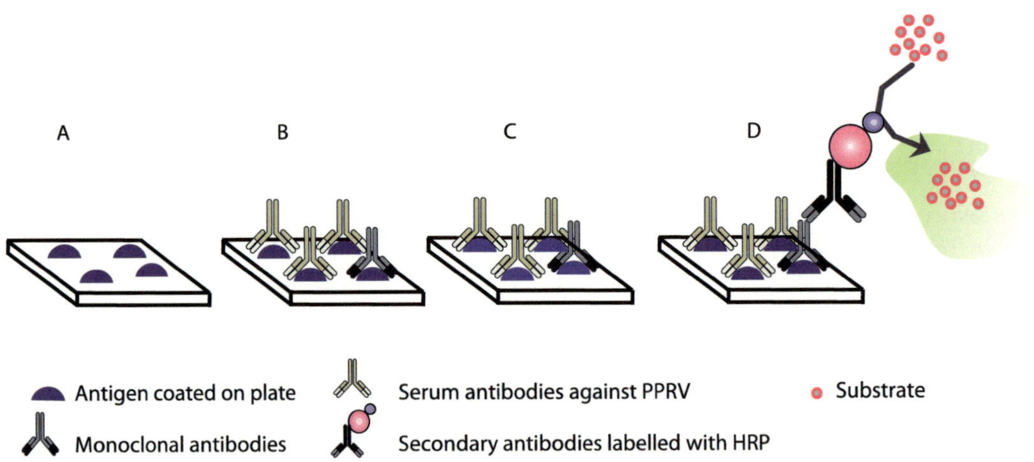

Fig. 4. Principle of competitive ELISA assays. (A) Coating the antigen on a polystyrene plate. (B) Addition of serum sample and monoclonal antibodies raised against the N protein of PPRV. (C) Addition of secondary antibodies labeled with enzyme. (D) Addition of substrate and reading the plate.

A competitive ELISA based on the use of MAb anti-nucleocapsid protein and a recombinant nucleocapsid protein produced in the baculovirus has been described (Libeau *et al.*, 1995; Libeau *et al.*, 1994).

1. Coat microtitre plates (e.g. high adsorption capacity NuncMaxisorb) with 50 µl of a predetermined dilution of N-PPR protein (produced by a recombinant baculovirus) for 1 hour at 37°C with constant agitation.
2. Wash the plates with washing solution (available in the kit) three times and blot dry.
3. Distribute 45 µl of blocking buffer (PBS + 0.5% Tween 20 + 0.5 fetal calf serum) to all wells, and then add 5 µl of test sera to test wells (at a final dilution of 1/20) and 5 µl of the different control sera (strong positive, weak positive and negative serum) to the control wells.
4. Add 50 µl of MAb diluted 1/100 in blocking buffer, and incubate at 37°C for 1 hour.
5. Wash the plates three times and blot dry.
6. Add 50 µl of anti-mouse conjugate diluted 1/1000, and incubate at 37°C for 1 hour.
7. Wash the plates three times.
8. Prepare OPD in hydrogen peroxide solution. Add 50 µl of substrate/conjugate mixture to each well.
9. Stop the reaction after 10 minutes with 50 µl of 1 M sulphuric acid.
10. Read on an ELISA reader at 492 nm.
    The absorbance is converted to percentage inhibition (PI) using the formula:
    PI=100-Absorbance of the test wells/Absorbance of the MAb control wells ×100
11. Sera showing PI greater than 50% are positive.

Another competitive ELISA technique, based on the use of monoclonal anti-haemagglutinin (H), has also been described (Choi *et al.*, 2005a).

5.5 Indirect immunofluorescence

The immunofluorescent antibody technique (IFA) has been practiced for rapid diagnosis of several pathogens including viruses and bacteria (Munir, 2011; Sumption *et al.*, 1998). However, if IFA is to play a reliable part in diagnostic virology then it is necessary to show that the results obtained are confirmed by the established procedures. This technique has been used to detect the PPRV antigen in conjunctival smears.

Principally, IFA is a technique allowing the visualization of a specific protein or antigen in cells or tissue sections by binding a specific antibody chemically conjugated with a fluorescent dye such as fluorescein isothiocyanate (FITC).

There are two major types of immunofluorescence staining methods:

1. Direct immunofluorescence staining in which the primary antibody is labeled with fluorescence dye, and
2. Indirect immunofluorescence staining in which a secondary antibody labeled with fluorochrome is used to recognize a primary antibody. Immunofluorescence staining can be performed on cells fixed on slides and tissue sections. Immunofluorescence stained samples are examined under a fluorescence microscope or confocal microscope. Due to this requirement of microscopy it is hard to apply this technique under field conditions.

5.6 Immunofiltration test

Immunofiltration (IF) assay is based on the surface adsorption of the antigen on the nitrocellulose membrane, and subsequent detection. Mainly, IF has been applied for the semiquantitative and/or qualitative detection of a wide range of pathogens. Since its development, IF has replaced several of the other immunoassays. The main advantage of the IF principle is its application in field conditions, and it can be taken as pen side test. Recently, IF has been employed for the detection of PPRV and compared with antigen-competition ELISA (AC-ELISA) (Raj *et al.*, 2008). It was proposed that IF is the best in screening larger samples in the field, and AC-ELISA can be used to confirm the important samples (Munir, 2011)

5.7 *In situ* immuno-peroxidase immunohistochemistry

A commercial streptavidin/biotin immunoperoxidase kit (LSAB 2 system, HRP, DacoCytomation, Denmark) can be used for this purpose. Tissue sections are digested with Proteinase K (0.1%) and incubated with a rabbit antirinderpest antibody (Institute for Animal Health, Pirbright, UK) at a dilution of 1/500. An aminoethylcarbazolechromogen substrate system (Labvision Corp., Fremont, CA) is applied for color reaction. Peste des petits ruminants virus positive tissues, previously confirmed with RT-PCR, are used as positive controls. Immunoperoxidase scoring is done on the basis of positively stained cells observed in 3 different areas at 403 microscope objective. The scores should be as follows: 0 (none): absent, 1+ (mild): a few immunopositive cells, 2+ (moderate): focal prominent Immuno-positivity, and 3+ (intense): strong immunopositivity in more than 50% of the cells.

5.8 Agar Gel Immunodiffusion test

Agar gel immunodiffusion (AGID) is a very simple and inexpensive test that can be performed in any laboratory and even in the field. Standard PPR viral antigen is prepared from mesenteric or bronchial lymph nodes, spleen or lung material and ground up as 1/3 suspensions in buffered saline. These are centrifuged at 500 g for 10–20 minutes, and the supernatant fluids are stored in aliquots at -20°C. The cotton material from the cotton bud used to collect eye or nasal swabs is removed using a scalpel and inserted into a 1 ml syringe. With 0.2 ml of phosphate buffered saline (PBS), the sample is extracted by repeatedly expelling and filling the 0.2 ml of PBS into an Eppendorf tube using the syringe plunger. The resulting eye/nasal swab extracted sample, like the tissue ground material prepared above, may be stored at -20°C until used. They may be retained for 1–3 years. Negative control antigen is prepared similarly from normal tissues. Standard antiserum is made by hyperimmunising sheep with 1 ml of PPRV with a titre of 104 TCID50 (50% tissue culture infective dose) per ml given at weekly intervals for 4 weeks. The animals are bled 5-7 days after the last injection (Munir *et al.*, 2009b; Osman *et al.*, 2008).

1. Dispense 1% agar in normal saline, containing thiomersal (0.4 g/litre) or sodium azide (1.25 g/litre) as a bacteriostatic agent, into Petri dishes (6 ml/5 cm dish).
2. Wells are punched in the agar following a hexagonal pattern with a central well. The wells are 5 mm in diameter and 5 mm apart.
3. The central well is filled with positive antiserum, three peripheral wells with positive antigen, and one well with negative antigen. The two remaining peripheral wells are filled with test antigen, such that the test and negative control antigens alternate with the positive control antigens.
4. Usually, 1–3 precipitin lines will develop between the serum and antigens within 18–24 hours (10).

5. These are intensified by washing the agar with 5% glacial acetic acid for 5 minutes (this procedure should be carried out with all apparently negative tests before recording a negative result). Positive reactions show lines of identity with the positive control antigen.
6. Results are obtained in one day, but the test is not sensitive enough to detect mild forms of PPR due to the low quantity of viral antigen that is excreted.

5.9 Counter Immunoelectrophoresis

Counter immunoelectrophoresis (CIEP) is the most rapid test for viral antigen detection. However, it has been applied for the serological detection of PPRV with as certain level of satisfaction (Munir *et al.*, 2009a). It is carried out on a horizontal surface using a suitable electrophoresis bath, which consists of two compartments connected through a bridge. The apparatus is connected to a high-voltage source. Agar or agarose (1–2%, [w/v]) dissolved in 0.025 M barbitone acetate buffer is dispensed onto microscope slides in 3-ml volumes. From six to nine pairs of wells are punched in the solidified agar. The reagents are the same as those used for the AGID test. The electrophoresis bath is filled with 0.1 M barbitone acetate buffer. The pairs of wells in the agar are filled with the reactants: sera in the anodal wells and antigen in the cathodal wells. The slide is placed on the connecting bridge and the ends are connected to the buffer in the troughs by wetted porous paper. The apparatus is covered, and a current of 10–12 milliamps per slide is applied for 30–60 minutes.

The current is switched off and the slides are viewed by intense light: the presence of 1–3 precipitation lines between pairs of wells is a positive reaction. There should be no reactions between wells containing the negative controls (Munir, 2011).

5.10 Nucleic acid detection of PPRV

There has been a substantial improvement in the detection of nucleic acid of PPRV in recent years. Demonstration of several real-time PCR assays have provided powerful and novel means of not only detection but also quantification of PPRV nucleic acids in several kinds of clinical samples. However, on the other side, these diagnostic tools are not readily available in all diagnostic laboratories especially in developing nations. There is a need to establish reliable, sensitive and affordable diagnostic tools that will be promptly accessible at low cost, independent of laboratory type. Therefore, there has been a strong tendency to increase the number of diagnostic tools based on diverse principles. While doing so, it is extremely important to design these assays in a way that these will be requiring less time, should be readily available, affordable for developing nations, not require high-tech facilities in laboratories, and must not be complex while performing under field conditions.

6. DIVA for PPRV and RP

The currently used live attenuated vaccine, using lineage I African isolate Nigeria 75/1, provides strong projection for at least three years. This vaccine, however, has certain limitations, including requirement for cold-chain maintenance, and inability to differentiate vaccinated from infected animals (DIVA). Development of such a technique would provide a practical and useful means to control the disease, especially in tropical countries. Research in several laboratories is in progress to produce a recombinant marker vaccine carrying either positive marker (addition of irrelevant B epitope), or negative marker (suppression of an epitope), with primary focus on serologically differentiating PPRV from RP.

7. Potential and need for future advances in serodiagnosis of PPR

Some of the conventional diagnostic serological methods that are currently available are rather time consuming, labour intensive and expensive. As the ultimate goal is to eradicate PPRV, as has been successfully done with RPV, the diagnostic methods that aid this goal have to be reliable, simple and quite cheap. They also need to work reliably during field conditions. As a vaccination strategy will be part of the eradication efforts, some kind of DIVA approach will be necessary. Also, the methods need to work independent of the genetic variants of PPRV that may exist. There is no doubt that the technology development in the field of diagnostic methods will expand fast. We have seen this especially in the nucleic acid detection field. Many methods can detect extremely small quantities of viral nucleic acid, down to one copy per PCR reaction. At this point it is difficult to judge what kind of technology to detect antibodies against PPRV will be the one that will be developed and accepted globally, if any. Probably, several types will be developed, tested and used in parallel, since many academic and corporate laboratories are working on this intensively. Usually, most technologies that are developed are too high tech to be accepted in routine diagnostic laboratories, and it takes some time to replace the already existing ones.

It is likely that we will have a combination of a simple field test device, such as a "dip-stick" that detects antibodies against PPRV, and possibly also some kind of vaccine marker. This can be used in combination with a simple field PCR machine, also with possibilities to differentiate between vaccinated and infected animals. In reference laboratories more advanced serological methods can be used, probably in combination with some kind of nucleic acid detection method.

In the more advanced reference laboratories flow cytometric bead-based technology has been successfully introduced, especially in human medicine. This technology will add new approaches that open up possibilities for simultaneous measurement of multiple molecules in samples. This relatively new technology allows for: (1) evaluation of multiple molecules in a single sample; (2) extremely small sample volumes; (3) high reproducibility; (4) direct comparison with existing assays; and finally (5) a more rapid evaluation of multiple samples in a single platform. For example, one can measure both IgG and IgM to be able to judge recent versus early infection, in combination with some key cytokines to determine the status of the infection, or even if this is a vaccinated animal, or vaccinated and infected in spite of the vaccination. Similarly, other pathogens can be tested simultaneously. However, at present the method needs rather expensive equipment and reagents; but we envision that this will become cheaper in the future.

8. Quality assurance in diagnostic laboratories

The veterinary diagnostic laboratories provide strategic support to field veterinarian, veterinary clinical services and public decision makers in controlling the important animal diseases. However, these activities can benefit veterinary services and public health only if the results produced by the laboratories are reliable, reproducible and rapid enough to be useful.

In many countries, veterinary diagnostic laboratories have not been able to contribute optimally to the community development because of: lack of clearly defined national policies for the laboratory services; shortage of qualified manpower; inappropriate laboratory equipment; poor development of internal quality control methods; and insufficient external quality assessment.

Today, providing funding for quality assurance should not been viewed only as a cost for the laboratories, but as an investment in building a permanent infrastructure and the competitive advantage for the laboratory, not only nationally but also internationally, in order to be able to respond to new animal health threats.

Setting up a quality assurance system in a veterinary diagnostic laboratory includes defining the structure, responsibilities, standard operating procedures and resources necessary to prevent the risks, to correct the errors and improve the efficiency of the laboratory, to ensure the quality of the results. One of the first steps to assure quality in laboratory practice is to conduct an assessment of laboratory systems. The quality assurance system comprises two types of activities: internal quality control that includes appropriate measures taken during day-to-day activities to control all possible variables that can influence the outcome of laboratory results: and external quality assessment to ensure comparability of results among laboratories.

A veterinary diagnostic laboratory working with diagnosis of PPRV should have the necessary staff with appropriate education and experience to carry out all the functions and responsibilities required from the personnel in a safe and accurate manner. This process should include not only management and scientific personnel but also administrative support, maintenance, cleaning and service team. All the staff should have a job description including: functions and responsibilities, academic training required and experience necessary.

The head of the laboratory must play the role of supervisor and motivator in ensuring quality of the results of the laboratory, and strive for continuous quality improvement throughout the organization.

9. Personal preparedness

The fundamental objective of the human resources policy should be to have competent staff with the scientific and/or appropriate technical training to apply appropriate laboratory procedures correctly. Staffing levels should be adequate to enable all the functions expected of the laboratory to be carried out without compromising safety the personal or the integrity of the processes performed in the laboratory.

PPRV is not known to infect humans in either laboratory or field settings. However, all of the personnel working with the potentially PPRV infected materials should wear protective clothing at all times for work in the laboratory; it is prohibited to wear laboratory clothing in any places outside the laboratory. Protective laboratory clothing that has been used in the laboratory must not be stored in the same lockers or cupboards as street clothing. Appropriate gloves must be worn for all procedures that may involve direct or accidental contact with specimens. After use, gloves should be removed aseptically and hands must then be washed. Personnel must wash their hands before they leave the laboratory working areas. Eating, drinking, smoking and applying cosmetics are prohibited in the laboratory working areas.

The greatest risk of working with PPRV is the escape of the organism into a susceptible animal population. Personnel who are working directly with potentially infected material should therefore strictly follow the measures necessary to minimize the risk of spreading the virus to the susceptible animals. Due to the highly contagious nature of the agent and the severe economic consequences of disease, laboratory workers should have no contact with susceptible hosts for five days after working with the agent.

There are specialized activities within the laboratory that require staff with considerable experience, such as ELISA techniques, cell culture production and virus isolation in cell culture, and RT-PCR and sequencing techniques. The laboratory must develop a continuing education program and regularly arrange training courses to update the skills of both technical and scientific staff according to needs identified by the management. This training is offered as a means of contributing to the success of the quality assurance process. The staff-training program should be documented to allow the correction of errors or weaknesses, and can also be used as a tool for promotion and follow-up of the performance of each staff member based on the job description.

10. Role and function of the laboratory in PPRV control and prevention

Although a tentative diagnosis of PPR can be proffered based on clinical signs, laboratory confirmation is required for differential diagnosis from other diseases with similar signs. Disease severity and the clinical signs depend on various factors: PPRV lineage, species, breed, immune status of animals. So a definitive diagnosis of PPRV infection cannot be based on clinical impressions alone, but must rely on laboratory confirmation. Detection of PPRV specific antibodies in serum is the standard test for the rapid laboratory diagnosis of PPRV. Antibody testing is most commonly performed using commercial enzyme linked immunoassay (ELISA) kits. Systems for the direct detection of PPRV through RT-PCR are becoming more common and, although standard methods are becoming established, no single standard method has yet been developed. Although not recommended for routine laboratory diagnosis, culture of PPR virus from clinical specimens is an important component of disease control strategies.

11. Structure and activities of the laboratory

The veterinary diagnostic laboratory dealing with PPRV should have adequate space to safely perform all activities, store all necessary equipment, and allow for easy cleaning and maintenance. Laboratory manipulation of clinical specimens for PPRV detection and identification, and serologic testing, are all associated with potential risks. These risks must be recognized and appropriate safety measures taken to prevent spread of the disease from the laboratory. Ideally all activities involving handling of infectious and potentially infectious diagnostic materials should take place in a limited access area under biosafety level 2 (BSL-2) conditions, and all activities involving the amplification of viruses, either in vitro or in vivo, should take place under BSL-3 conditions.

Staff working with the live viruses must undergo appropriate training, in order to minimize risk to laboratory staff and spread of the virus outside the laboratory. All laboratory procedures using infectious or potentially infectious materials must be carried out in a fully functioning Biological Safety Cabinet (a ventilated laboratory workspace for safely working with materials contaminated with pathogens requiring a defined biosafety level). Cabinets must be adequately maintained and periodically tested for correct operation. All pipetting should be done using an automatic or manual safety pipetting device; mouth pipetting must not be permitted. Improper handling of the cell cultures must be avoided. Any laboratory accident should be reported to a supervisor *immediately* for the further action to minimize the effect of the accident.

There should be enough rooms to enable separation of infectious from non-infectious activities, to minimize the chances of contamination of clean areas. Lighting and ventilation should correspond to the needs of each working area, according to the specific requirements of the activity carried out. The surfaces of the workbenches should be smooth, easy to clean and made of material resistant to chemicals. Cell culture and media-making facilities should be separated from the laboratory where viral or other microbiological activities are being carried out. If space allows, specific areas and preferably specific rooms should be allocated for:

1. Reagents and consumables storage;
2. Instruments and equipment;
3. Specimen receipt and recording;
4. Specimen processing;
5. Serology;
6. Cell culture;
7. Virus handling;
8. Specialized activities;
9. Documentation and archiving;
10. The administrative area; and
11. Disposal of contaminated wastes.

12. Equipment and instruments

The laboratory should have the necessary equipment and instruments for the accurate performance of all tests to be performed. Before installation of equipment and organization of the laboratories biosafety and other safety standards should be take into account. New instruments and equipment should be installed and calibrated if possible by the qualified person. All manuals and operating instructions should be stored in an area accessible to all users, and a regular maintenance and calibration schedule must be established. All users must be undergoing an introduction in order to be fully familiar with the operation, maintenance and validation procedures to ensure correct functioning of the equipment. Documentation of all malfunctions, maintenance and validation activities should be recorded. The laboratory should have a list of equipment and instruments that include:

1. The name;
2. Brand;
3. Supplier;
4. Maintenance company;
5. Maintenance schedule;

6. Inventory number;
7. Serial number;
8. Model and year;
9. Location;
10. Date of purchase; and
11. Copy of manufacturer's handbook.

13. Supplies

13.1 Reference materials

These include materials such as reference positive and negative control sera, used for calibration of the test procedures. Reference materials are also used to guarantee uniformity in determining activity. These materials should be purchased from certified suppliers, and purchasing, reception and distribution must be the responsibility of a qualified professional. A central record should be kept with the name of the reference material, supplier, and origin and lot number.

This registry should contain all the information relating to the properties of the reference material. The quality of the reference material should be verified when the conditions have been altered, and routinely once a year.

13.2 Reagents (including diagnostic kits)

These can be defined as materials of chemical or biological origin used in laboratory assays. Because of difficulty of transport to some regions, reagents should be ordered some months ahead of need. The reagents should be of appropriate quality and be obtained from recommended suppliers. A record should be kept of purchasing, reception and distribution to guarantee continuity, particularly with substances that need to be acquired in advance.

Reagents prepared in the laboratory should be prepared in conformity with written procedures and, where applicable, according to OIE/FAO standard recommendations, validated and labeled appropriately, stating the following:

1. Identification of the reagent;
2. Concentration;
3. Preparation and expiry date;
4. Storage conditions;
5. Initials of the technician responsible.

13.3 Laboratory safety

Each laboratory should have available a safety policy document that describes the essential biosafety, chemical, fire and electrical safety requirements to protect staff, the community and the environment. The content of this document should be well implemented in the daily work of the staff, and all the personnel should be familiar with the contents of the safety policy document and should proceed accordingly. All new staff should be made aware of the risks involved in working in a laboratory before starting work in the laboratory. The head of the laboratory is responsible for implementation of and compliance with the provisions of the safety policy document.

The major risk to staff in the laboratory is in handling the clinical samples. The clinical samples should always be considered as a potentially infectious material, and personnel should wear gloves when opening packages containing the clinical samples, aliquoting or transferring samples and when performing assays. Personnel who receive and unpack specimens should be aware of the potential health hazards involved, and should be trained to adopt standard precautions, particularly when dealing with broken or leaking containers. Primary specimen containers should be opened in a biological safety cabinet where possible. Disinfectants should be available in case of spills.

14. Annexes

14.1 Example for PPRV laboratory request form

Sample submission form

Basic Information

Sender name:............ Name of sender lab:............

Date of sample collection:............ Sample ID:............

Demographic Information

Name, address, location of the owener:............

Total animals in a herd:............ goats are:............sheep are:............

Species: Goat:............ Sheep:............

Breed:............ Age:............

Sex:............

Disease Information

Diseased animals are:............ Dead animals are:............ Aborted animals are:............

Health Status: Very good............Good............Poor............Very poor............

Previous treatment to any disease:............

PPRV vaccination: Yes............No............

Specimen Information

Whole Blood :............ Oral Mucosa .... Lungs............ Brain............
Serum .... Tonsils............ Liver .... Kidney............
Swab .... Spleen .... Intestine............

Clinical signs of the disease

Abortion............
Diarrhea............
Pneumonia............
Oral mucosa lesions ....
Parasitism ....
Other (please specify)
....

Management of the herd

Housing............
Nutrition............
Feeding............
Other (please specify)
....

Signature............

14.2 Composition of media and reagents

14.2.1 Phosphate Buffered Saline (PBS)

To prepare 1 liter (L) of PBS, the following reagents will be required:

Reagents	Quantity
Sodium chloride NaCl	8g
Potassium chloride KCl	0.2g
Potassium dihydrogen phosphate anhydrous KH_2PO_4	0.2g
Disodium hydrogen phosphate anhydrous Na_2HPO_4 **OR**	0.92g
Disodium hydrogen phosphate dihydrous $Na_2HPO_4.2H_2O$ **OR**	1.15g
Disodium hydrogen phosphate dodecahydrous $Na_2HPO_4.12H_2O$	2.32g
Distilled water to make up to 1 L	QS

1. Weigh all the reagents and add to a 5 L conical flask.
2. Add distilled water to make 1 L and mix well.
3. Adjust the pH to 7.3 to 7.4.
4. Pour into storage bottles.
5. Autoclave at 121°C and 15 pound per square inch (psi) for 15 minutes. Use a slow exhaust.
6. Allow cooling, then tighten the lids and label the bottles.

Similarly, a greater concentration or volume of PBS can be prepared.

14.2.2 Preparation of 1% nobal agar

To prepare 1% nobal agar, the following reagents will be required.

Reagents	Quantity
Nobal agar	1g
Tris-Borate EDTA (TBE) buffer	1L

1. Weigh 1 gram of nobal agar and add to 1 L of Tris-Borate EDTA (TBE) buffer in a 2 L Erlenmeyer flask.
2. Mix the agar until it dissolve and autoclave the mixture for 10 minutes. Continuously stir the contents by swirling to ensure a homogeneous mixture of ingredients after removing from the autoclave. After autoclaving, allow the agar to cool at room temperature (approximately 25°C) and 15 psi for 10 to 15 minutes before dispensing into Petri plates.
3. Dispence the agar into small quantities (daily working volumes) and store in airtight containers at 4°C for several weeks. These working flasks can be melted and dispensed into plates as needed.

NOTE: Agar or agar plates cannot be used if microbial contamination or precipitate are observed.

15. References

Abraham, G. & Berhan, A. (2001). The use of antigen-capture enzyme-linked immunosorbent assay (ELISA) for the diagnosis of rinderpest and peste des petits ruminants in ethiopia. *Tropical animal health and production* 33(5), 423-30.

Abubakar, M., Jamal, S.M., Hussain, M. & Ali, Q. (2008). Incidence of peste des petits ruminants (PPR) virus in sheep and goat as detected by immuno-capture ELISA (Ic ELISA). *Small ruminants research* 75, 256-259.

Abubakar, M., Rajput, Z.I., Arshed, M.J., Sarwar, G. & Ali, Q. (2011). Evidence of peste des petits ruminants virus (PPRV) infection in Sindh Ibex (Capra aegagrus blythi) in Pakistan as confirmed by detection of antigen and antibody. *Tropical animal health and production* 43(4), 745-7.

Anderson, J. & McKay, J.A. (1994). The detection of antibodies against peste des petits ruminants virus in cattle, sheep and goats and the possible implications to rinderpest control programmes. *Epidemiology and infection* 112(1), 225-31.

Anderson, J., McKay, J.A. & Butcher, R.N. (1991). *The use of monoclonal antibodies in competition ELISA for detection of antibodies to rinderpest and peste des petits ruminants viruses. In: The Seromonitoring of Rinderpest Throughout Africa: Phase I.*: IAEA, Vienna, Austria.

Aslam, M., Abubakar, M., Anjum, R., Saleha, S. & Ali, Q. (2009). Prevalence of Peste Des Petits Ruminants Virus (PPRV) in Mardan, Hangu and Kohat District of Pakistan; Comparative Analysis of PPRV Suspected serum samples using Competitive ELISA (cELISA) and Agar Gel Immunodiffusion (AGID). *Veterinary world* 2(3), 89-92.

Atta-ur-Rahman, Ashfaque, M., Rahman, S.U., Akhtar, M. & Ullah, S. (2004). Peste des petits ruminants antigen in mesenteric lymph nodes of goats slaughtered at D. I. Khan. *Pakistan veterinary journal* 24(3), 159-160.

Bailey, D., Banyard, A., Dash, P., Ozkul, A. & Barrett, T. (2005). Full genome sequence of peste des petits ruminants virus, a member of the Morbillivirus genus. *Virus research* 110(1-2), 119-24.

Banyard, A.C., Parida, S., Batten, C., Oura, C., Kwiatek, O. & Libeau, G. (2010). Global distribution of peste des petits ruminants virus and prospects for improved diagnosis and control. *Journal of general virology* 91(Pt 12), 2885-97.

Barrett, T, Pastoret P.P & Taylor W.P. (2005). Rinderpest and Peste Des Petits Ruminants: Virus Plagues of Large and Small Ruminants Eds. Elsevier Academic Press.

Bodjo, S.C., Kwiatek, O., Diallo, A., Albina, E. & Libeau, G. (2007). Mapping and structural analysis of B-cell epitopes on the morbillivirus nucleoprotein amino terminus. *Journal of general virology* 88(Pt 4), 1231-42.

Brindha, K., Raj, G.D., Ganesan, P.I., Thiagarajan, V., Nainar, A.M. & Nachimuthu, K. (2001). Comparison of virus isolation and polymerase chain reaction for diagnosis of peste des petits ruminants. *Acta virologica* 45(3), 169-72.

Bruning-Richardson, A., Akerblom, L., Klingeborn, B. & Anderson, J. (2011). Improvement and development of rapid chromatographic strip-tests for the diagnosis of rinderpest and peste des petits ruminants viruses. *Journal of virological methods* 174(1-2), 42-6.

Choi, K.S., Nah, J.J., Ko, Y.J., Kang, S.Y. & Jo, N.I. (2005a). Rapid competitive enzyme-linked immunosorbent assay for detection of antibodies to peste des petits ruminants virus. *Clinical and diagnostic laboratory immunology* 12(4), 542-7.

Choi, K.S., Nah, J.J., Ko, Y.J., Kang, S.Y., Yoon, K.J. & Jo, N.I. (2005b). Antigenic and immunogenic investigation of B-cell epitopes in the nucleocapsid protein of peste des petits ruminants virus. *Clinical and diagnostic laboratory immunology* 12(1), 114-21.

Diallo, A., Libeau, G., Couacy-Hymann, E. & Barbron, M. (1995). Recent developments in the diagnosis of rinderpest and peste des petits ruminants. *Veterinary microbiology* 44(2-4), 307-17.

Diallo, A., Minet, C., Le Goff, C., Berhe, G., Albina, E., Libeau, G. & Barrett, T. (2007). The threat of peste des petits ruminants: progress in vaccine development for disease control. *Vaccine* 25(30), 5591-7.

Diop, M., Sarr, J. & Libeau, G. (2005). Evaluation of novel diagnostic tools for peste des petits ruminants virus in naturally infected goat herds. *Epidemiology and infection* 133(4), 711-7.

Ezeibe, M.C., Okoroafor, O.N., Ngene, A.A., Eze, J.I., Eze, I.C. & Ugonabo, J.A. (2008). Persistent detection of peste de petits ruminants antigen in the faeces of recovered goats. *Tropical animal health and production* 40(7), 517-9.

Furley, C.W., Taylor, W.P. & Obi, T.U. (1987). An outbreak of peste des petits ruminants in a zoological collection. *The veterinary record* 121(19), 443-7.

Gargadennec, L & Lalanne, A. (1942) La peste des petits ruminants. *Bulletin des Services Zootechniques et des Epizooties de I'Afrique Occidntale Francaise* 5, 16–21.

Gibbs, E.P.J., Taylor, W.P., Lawman, M.P.J. & Bryant, J. (1979). Classification of the peste-despetits-ruminants virus as the fourth member of the genus Morbillivirus. *Intervirology* 11, 268–274.

Hussain, M., Muneer, R., Jahangir, M., Awan, A.H., Khokhar, M.A., Zahur, A.B., Zulfiqar, M. & Hussain, A. (2003). Chromatographic strip technology: a pen-side test for the rapid diagnosis of peste des petits ruminants in sheep and goats. *Journal of biological sciences* 3, 1-7.

Ismail, I.M. & House, J. (1990). Evidence of identification of peste des petits ruminants from goats in Egypt. *Archiv fur experimentelle veterinarmedizin* 44(3), 471-4.

Keerti, M., Sarma, B.J. & Reddy, Y.N. (2009). Development and application of latex agglutination test for detection of PPR virus. *Indian Veterinary Journal* 86, 234-237.

Khan, H.A., Siddique, M., Arshad, M.J., Khan, Q.M. & Rehman, S.U. (2007). Sero-prevalence of peste des petits ruminants (PPR) virus in sheep and goats in Punjab province of Pakistan. *Pakistan veterinary journal* 27(3), 109-112.

Kitching, R.P. (1988). *The economic significance and control of small ruminant viruses in North Africa and West Asia. In Increasing small ruminant productivity in semi-arid areas.*: Kluwer Academic Publishers-Dordrecht. The Netherlands.

Libeau, G., Diallo, A., Colas, F. & Guerre, L. (1994). Rapid differential diagnosis of rinderpest and peste des petits ruminants using an immunocapture ELISA. *Veterinary record* 134(12), 300-4.

Libeau, G., Prehaud, C., Lancelot, R., Colas, F., Guerre, L., Bishop, D.H. & Diallo, A. (1995). Development of a competitive ELISA for detecting antibodies to the peste des petits ruminants virus using a recombinant nucleoprotein. *Research in veterinary science* 58(1), 50-5.

Mahapatra, M., Parida, S., Baron, M.D. & Barrett, T. (2006). Matrix protein and glycoproteins F and H of Peste-des-petits-ruminants virus function better as a homologous complex. *The journal of general virology* 87(Pt 7), 2021-9.

Manoharan, S., Jayakumar, R., Govindarajan, R. and Koteeswaran, A. 2005 (2005). Haemagglutination as a confirmatory test for Peste des petits ruminants diagnosis. 59(75-78).

Munir, M. (2011). Diagnosis of Peste des Petits Ruminants under limited resource setting: A cost effective strategy for developing countries where PPRV is endemic. 1st. ed: VDM Verlag Dr. Müller.

Munir, M., Abubakar, M., Khan, M.T. & Abro, S.H. (2009a). Comparative efficacy of single radial haemolysis test and countercurrent immunoelectro-osmophoresis with monoclonal antibodies-based competitive ELISA for the serology of Peste des Petits Ruminants in Sheep and Goats. *Bulgarian journal of veterinary medicine* 12(4), 246-253.

Munir, M., Siddique, M. & Ali, Q. (2009b). Comparative efficacy of standard AGID and precipitinogen inhibition test with monoclonal antibodies based competitive ELISA for the serology of Peste des Petits Ruminants in sheep and goats. *Tropical animal health and production* 41(3), 413-20.

Munir, M., Zohari, S., Saeed, A., Khan, Q.M., Abubakar, M., Leblanc, N. & Berg, M. (2011). Detection and Phylogenetic Analysis of Peste des Petits Ruminants Virus Isolated from Outbreaks in Punjab, Pakistan. *Transboundary and emerging diseases DOI: 10.1111/j.1865-1682.2011.01245.x.*

Obi, T.U. & Ojeh, C.K. (1989). Dot enzyme immunoassay for visual detection of peste-des-petits-ruminants virus antigen from infected caprine tissues. *Journal of clinical microbiology* 27(9), 2096-9.

Obi, T.U. & Patrick, D. (1984). The detection of peste des petits ruminants (PPR) virus antigen by agar gel precipitation test and counter-immunoelectrophoresis. *The Journal of hygiene* 93(3), 579-86.

OIE (2008). *Peste des petits ruminants. Chapter 2.7.11. In Manual of diagnostic tests and vaccines for terrestrial animal health.* 6th. ed: Office International des Epizooties/World Organization for Animal Health (OIE), Paris I and II).

Osman, N.A., ME, A.R., Ali, A.S. & Fadol, M.A. (2008). Rapid detection of Peste des Petits Ruminants (PPR) virus antigen in Sudan by agar gel precipitation (AGPT) and haemagglutination (HA) tests. *Tropical animal health and production* 40(5), 363-8.

Perl, S., Alexander, A., Yacobson, B., Nyska, A., Harmelin, A., Sheikhat, N., Shimshony, A., Davidson, M., Abramson, M. & Rapaport, E. (1995). Peste des petits ruminants (PPR) of sheep in Israel: case report. *Israel journal of veterinary medicine* 49(59-62).

Rabenau H., Kessler H.H., Kortenbusch M., Steinhorst A., Raggam R.B. & Berger A. (2007). Verification and validation of diagnostic laboratory tests in clinical virology. *Journal of clinical virology* 40, 93–98.

Raj, G.D., Rajanathan, T.M., Kumar, C.S., Ramathilagam, G., Hiremath, G. & Shaila, M.S. (2008). Detection of peste des petits ruminants virus antigen using immunofiltration and antigen-competition ELISA methods. *Veterinary microbiology* 129(3-4), 246-51.

Renukaradhya, G.J., Sinnathamby, G., Seth, S., Rajasekhar, M. & Shaila, M.S. (2002). Mapping of B-cell epitopic sites and delineation of functional domains on the hemagglutinin-neuraminidase protein of peste des petits ruminants virus. *Virus research* 90(1-2), 171-85.

Saliki, J.T., Brown, C.C., House, J.A. & Dubovi, E.J. (1994). Differential immunohistochemical staining of peste des petits ruminants and rinderpest antigens in formalin-fixed, paraffin-embedded tissues using monoclonal and polyclonal antibodies. *Journal of veterinary diagnostic investigation* 6(1), 96-8.

Saravanan, P., Balamurugan, V., Sen, A., Bikash, B. & Singh, R.K. (2006). Development of dot ELISA for diagnosis of Peste des petits ruminants (PPR) in small ruminants. *Journal of Applied Animal Research* 30, 121-124.

Saravanan, P., Sen, A., Balamurugan, V., Bandyopadhyay, S.K. & Singh, R.K. (2008). Rapid quality control of a live attenuated Peste des petits ruminants (PPR) vaccine by monoclonal antibody based sandwich ELISA. *Biologicals* 36(1), 1-6.

Sen, A., Saravanan, P., Balamurugan, V., Rajak, K.K., Sudhakar, S.B., Bhanuprakash, V., Parida, S. & Singh, R.K. (2010). Vaccines against peste des petits ruminants virus. *Expert review of vaccines* 9(7), 785-96.

Seth, S. & Shaila, M.S. (2001). The hemagglutinin-neuraminidase protein of peste des petits ruminants virus is biologically active when transiently expressed in mammalian cells. *Virus research* 75(2), 169-77.

Shaila, M.S., Shamaki, D., Forsyth, M.A., Diallo, A., Goatley, L., Kitching, R.P. & Barrett, T. (1996). Geographic distribution and epidemiology of peste des petits ruminants virus. *Virus research* 43(2), 149-53.

Singh, R.P., Saravanan, P., Sreenivasa, B.P., Singh, R.K. & Bandyopadhyay, S.K. (2004). Prevalence and distribution of peste des petits ruminants virus infection in small ruminants in India. *Revue scientifique et technique* 23(3), 807-19.

Sreenivasa, B.P., Singh, R.P., Mondal, B., Dhar, P. & Bandyopadhyay, S.K. (2006). Marmoset B95a cells: a sensitive system for cultivation of Peste des petits ruminants (PPR) virus. *Veterinary research communications* 30(1), 103-8.

Sumption, K.J., Aradom, G., Libeau, G. & Wilsmore, A.J. (1998). Detection of peste des petits ruminants virus antigen in conjunctival smears of goats by indirect immunofluorescence. *The Veterinary record* 142(16), 421-4.

World Organization for Animal Health (2008). OIE *Terrestrial Manual* 2008; *Chapter 1.1.3. - Quality management in veterinary testing laboratories.* World Organization for Animal Health (OIE: Office International des Epizooties), 12 rue de Prony, 75017 Paris, France.

World Organization for Animal Health (2008). Standard for Management and Technical Requirements for Laboratories Conducting Tests for Infectious Animal Diseases. *In:* OIE Quality Standard and Guidelines for Veterinary Laboratories: Infectious Diseases, Second Edition. World Organisation for Animal Health (OIE: Office International des Epizooties), 12 rue de Prony, 75017 Paris, France, 1–25.

Wosu, L.O. (1985). Agglutination of red blood cells by peste des petits ruminants (PPR) virus. *Nigerian Veterinary Journal* 14, 56–58.

5

Some Selected Serological Diagnostic Techniques in Plant Virology

A. A. Fajinmi
Dept. of Crop Protection, COLPLANT,
Federal University of Agriculture Abeokuta,
Alabata, Ogun State,
Nigeria

1. Introduction

Particle morphology, host range and the serological properties of the coat protein are generally being used to identify plant viruses. In classification and the establishment of taxonomic relationships, cross-reactivity of antisera raised against viruses from different groups have been frequently used (KPL Technical Guide on line 1999/2000 edition). However sequence data of nucleic acid are accumulating rapidly and are allowing more accurate relationships to be established between the individual members of virus groups than serological methods do (Dellaporta *et al.* 1983; Jackie Hughes *et al* 2004). Sequencing parts of a virus genome is often done in the identification of a virus if detailed serological analysis cannot provide conclusive data about the virus (Dellaporta *et al.* 1983). This involves purification and isolation of the virus particles and the subsequent cloning of parts of the virus. Using advance molecular methods in specific Polymerase chain reaction (PCR), new virus sequence data can be obtained without the need to purify a virus or to clone parts of its genome (Jackie Hughes *et al* 2004). Advances in molecular biotechnology have contributed immensely in developing specific and sensitive diagnostic assays and sensitive antisera against individual viruses or group of viruses (Dellaporta *et al.* 1983; Jackie Hughes *et al* 2004). Useful tools are provided in diagnostic procedures for virus disease monitoring.

2. Virus diagnosis

Different diagnostic techniques are used in the identification of plant viruses. Symptom observations is an important tool in field virus diagnosis though it is not a conclusive methods, it is combined with other methods (Fajinmi, 2006). One of such methods is transmission studies, which involves studies on how a virus gets into host plants. Different indicator test plants are mechanically inoculated or graft transmitted with the virus, insect vector transmission of the virus are carried out on series of test plants in specialized insect proof cages so as to provide useful information and further characterizing the virus (Jackie Hughes *et al* 2004; Fajinmi, 2011). Environmental factors may influence the symptom expression of the virus which may serve as a limiting factor but the use of electron microscopy brings further clarification of the virus (Jackie Hughes *et al* 2004; Fajinmi, 2006; Fajinmi, 2011).

3. Types of serological tests

There are principally two types of serological test, the liquid phase test and the solid phase test (Jackie Hughes *et al* 2004). Both methods are basically interaction between known antibodies and the unknown virus for positive identification, but visualization differs. In liquid phase test, there is formation of a visible precipitate in a solution reaction, i.e. agglutination of visible cells. This kind of test include, gel diffusion test, precipitin or micro-precipitin test (Jackie Hughes *et al* 2004).

In solid phase test, it is an enzymatic reaction, where antibodies are conjugated with a marker enzyme in which the antibody attaches itself with the antigen after recognizing it (Jackie Hughes *et al* 2004). The chosen enzyme reacts with the substrate to provide a positive identification. This is confirmed through colour change in the substrate. Examples of this test include micro-titre plates or nitrocellulose membranes (Jackie Hughes *et al* 2004).

4. Test methods selection

Test method could be selected depending on the reason of the serological analysis, the information required and availability of materials to be used (Jackie Hughes *et al* 2004). Diagnosis is performed in optimum conditions with proper controls and must be reproducible. This will enhance proper, correct and desirable data analysis for the result to be valid. Availability of laboratory equipment and antibodies will determine the specific serological test to be used (Jackie Hughes *et al* 2004).

5. Serological techniques

5.1 Double diffusion tests

The materials needed to design, perform and evaluate double diffusion tests includes, (1) Pipette (10 µl - 100 µl is preferred; other pipettes can be used) (2) Flat bottomed glass or plastic dishes (Petri dishes are recommended) (3) Agar (4) phosphate Buffer (5) cork borer for punching out well patterns (6) tight sealed moist chamber for incubation with moist towel in bottom (Jackie Hughes *et al* 2004).

Test Procedure as described by Jackie Hughes *et al* (2004)

a. Dissolve 70mg of agar in 100mls of buffer (0.7 % W/V) and autoclave at 120°C for 10 minutes, Cool to 60° C.
b. Dispense to sterilized Petri-dishes and allow to fully solidify.
c. With the aid of a cork borer, punch out well patterns on the solidified agar in the Petri-dish with no damage to the clean - cut sides of the wells.
d. Dispense the antibodies and antigen to the wells according to the test pattern.
e. Incubate text plate in the moist chamber for 5-7 days.

6. Determination of optimum antigen/antibody concentrations

Optimum concentration for antigen and antibodies can be determined by creating a pattern of six wells in a circular pattern around one central well (Jackie Hughes *et al* 2004). The six wells are filled with different concentration of antibodies (double fold dilutions mg/ml). In another plate different concentration of antigen could be used (Jackie Hughes *et al* 2004). A thin sharp line of precipitation will be shown between the antigen well and the antibody well that is having the right concentration (Jackie Hughes *et al* 2004).

7. Interpreting double diffusion test results

There is a radial diffusion of the antigen and antibodies form the wells. Lines of precipitate are formed in the agar as the antibodies and antigen meet; results are interpreted based on these patterns of precipitate (Jackie Hughes *et al* 2004). Combination of antibodies and antigen must be properly balanced with the correct dilutions for correct interpretation (Jackie Hughes *et al* 2004).

8. Enzyme-Linked Immunosorbent Assay (ELISA) tests

This is the most common technique for diagnosing of plant viruses and it is a solid phase assay. The test reaction involves antibody and antigen reaction to produce a positive reaction. The reaction takes place in a microtitre plates made of either polystyrene or polyvinyl chloride (PVC) (KPL Technical Guide (on line 1999/2000 edition); Jackie Hughes *et al* (2004). Antibodies conjugated to a "marker enzyme" are used in ELISA. Reaction between the antibody and the antigen will make the "marker enzyme" to react in the substrate resulting in colour development (KPL Technical Guide on line 1999/2000 edition); Jackie Hughes *et al* 2004).

There is "direct" and "indirect" ELISA test. In "direct" ELISA test, the detecting antibody bounds with the marker enzyme while in "indirect" ELISA test, the antibody enzyme conjugate binds with the detecting primary antibody and not directly with the virus (KPL Technical Guide on line 1999/2000 edition); Jackie Hughes *et al.* 2004).

"Direct" ELISA procedure as described by KPL technical guide (on line 1999/2000 edition) and Jackie Hughes *et al* (2004)

Coat the microtitre plate with antibodies followed by the virus sample. The virus becomes bound to the antibodies for a positive reaction. Wash the plates with phosphate buffer in Tween-20 to remove any of the virus samples that has not reacted with the antibodies. Add antibody enzyme conjugates then wash again to remove excess unbound conjugate then add the substrate. Colour development provides and indication that the virus and the antibody have reacted. This shows that the antibody enzyme conjugates has attached to the trapped virus allowing the enzyme to react. This confirms a tentative virus identification and quantification. This test method is referred to as double antibody sand which (DAS) ELISA because the virus is sandwiched between the capturing antibody and the detecting antibody. This method is strain specific and the antibody to detect the virus must be conjugated to an enzyme and a specific conjugate is required for each antibody to be used.

"Indirect" ELISA

This involves the usage of antibodies which have been raised to two different animals and using different methods for capturing the virus (KPL Technical Guide on line 1999/2000 edition). Though the antibodies that identify with the virus have been raised for that specific virus, the secondary antibody marker can be raised to recognize a wide range of primary antibodies, with the fact that the primary antibodies were produced in the same animal species against which the secondary antibodies were raised (Jackie Hughes *et al* 2004). It is cheaper to produce a secondary marker antibody enzyme conjugate in "indirect" ELISA than primary marker antibody enzyme conjugate in "direct" ELISA (Jackie Hughes *et al* 2004). Two different animals are used in the production of primary and secondary antibodies (Jackie Hughes *et al* 2004). In recognizing specific viruses, primary antibodies are raised in one animal species, while production of secondary antibodies is to recognize proteins from specific species of animal (Jackie Hughes *et al* 2004). For instance, antibodies as protein source from rabbit can be used as antigen to produce secondary antibody from mouse (Jackie Hughes *et al* 2004). These secondary antibodies from mouse can bund with any antibodies produced in a rabbit.

Examples of "indirect" ELISA methods as described by KPL Technical Guide (on line 1999/2000 edition) and Jackie Hughes *et al* (2004) include; Antigen coated plate (ACP) or plate trapped (PTA), direct antigen coated (DAC) assays. In this assays, the first to be added is the primary antibodies, then the secondary antibody enzyme conjugate and substrate. In triple antibody sandwich (TAS) ELISA, three antibodies are used in a sequential order. Trapping antibodies followed by the virus sample then the primary antibodies added followed by the secondary enzyme conjugated antibodies which binds with the primary antibodies. Protein A sandwich (PAS) ELISA uses protein A for an increase in the test specific and reaction sensitivity by controlling orientation of antibodies. Steps involve; Plate covered with protein A → trapping antibodies →virus sample →secondary antibody. Protein A will detect by biding with the secondary antibodies if in correct orientation.

9. ELISA buffers

9.1 Phosphate buffered saline

8.0 g NaCl
0.2 g KH_2PO_4
1.1 g Na_2HPO_4
0.2 g KCL

(Add up to litre with distilled water)

9.2 PBS-tween

Add 0.5ml Tween 20 (0.05%v/v) to 999.5 ml PBS pH 7.4

9.3 Coating buffer pH 9.6

1.59 g Na_2CO_3
2.93 g $NaHCO_3$

(Add up to litre with distilled water)

9.4 Conjugate buffer

Half strength PBS containing
0.05% v/v Tween 20
0.02% w/v egg albumin (ovalbumen)
0.2% w/v polyvinylpyrrolidone (PVP)

9.5 Substrate buffer pH 9.8

97 ml diethanolamine
800 ml H_2O
Add HCL to give pH 9.8

(Add up to litre with distilled water)

Store all buffers at 4°C and monitor its pH before use. Buffers should be replaced if not used within one month.

Examples of ELISA Virus indexing protocols as described by KPL Technical Guide (on line 1999/2000 edition) and Jackie Hughes *et al* (2004)

Weigh 1 g of leaf sample in 3 ml of extraction buffer (PBS-Tween + 2% (w/v) Polyvinylpyrrolidone (PVP) in a sterilized mortar and grind with a sterile pestle in a circular motion to form a paste. Sieve supernatant by carefully removing the plant debris into sterile Eppendorf tube container.

Example protocols for Antigen Coated Plate (ACP) ELISA as described by KPL Technical Guide (on line 1999/2000 edition) and Jackie Hughes *et al* (2004).

1. Add 100µl of antigen ground in extraction buffer into plates
2. Cover plate and incubate over night at 4°C
3. Wash plate 3 times with PBS-Tween by flooding 3 times. Drain and tap plate dry
4. Block with 200µl per well of 3% (w/v) dried non fat skimmed milk in PBS-Tween
5. Cover plate and incubate at 37°C for 30 minutes
6. Empty and tap plate dry
7. Add 100µl per well of antibody (monoclonal or polyclonal) diluted in conjugate buffer 1:2000
8. Cover plate and incubate at 37°C for 2 hours
9. Wash plate 3 times with PBS-Tween by flooding for 3 times. Tap plate dry
10. Add 100µl per well of either goat anti mouse or goat anti-rabbit alkaline phosphate conjugate diluted in conjugate buffer 1:2000
11. Cover plate and incubate at 37°C for 2 hours
12. Wash plate 3 times with PBS-Tween by flooding for 3 times. Tap plate dry
13. Add 200µl per well of 0.5- 1 mg/ml of p-nitrophenyl phosphate substrate in substrate buffer.
14. Read the plate after 1 hour and or overnight.

Example protocols for Protein - A sandwich (PAS) ELISA as described by KPL Technical Guide (on line 1999/2000 edition) and Jackie Hughes *et al* (2004).

1. Add 100µl of protein A per well in extraction buffer into plates

2. Cover plate and incubate the plates at 37°C for 2 hours
3. Wash plate 3 times with PBS-Tween by flooding 3 times. Drain and tap plate dry
4. Grind virus free leaf sample in PBS-Tween at a dilution of 1:5
5. Dilute the antiserum 1: 2000 in virusfree leaf extract and incubate for 20-30 minutes at 37°C to cross-adsorbed any antibodies to plant proteins.
6. Add 100µl per well of cross-adsorbed polyclonal antiserum to each well
7. Cover plate and incubate at 37°C for 2 hours
8. Wash plate 3 times with PBS-Tween by flooding 3 times. Drain and tap plate dry
9. Add 100 µl of antigen (virus sample) ground in PBS-Tween + 2% PVP
10. Cover plate and incubate overnight at 4°C
11. Wash plate 3 times with PBS-Tween by flooding 3 times. Drain and tap plate dry
12. Add 100 µl of diluted (as in step 5) and cross-adsorbed polyclonal antiserum
13. Cover plate and incubate at 37°C for 2 hours
14. Wash plate 3 times with PBS-Tween by flooding 3 times. Drain and tap plate dry
15. Add 100 µl per well of Protein A Alkaline phosphate conjugate at a dilution of 1:1000 in conjugate buffer
16. Cover plate and incubate at 37°C for 2 hours
17. Wash plate 3 times with PBS-Tween by flooding 3 times. Drain and tap plate dry
18. Add 200 µl per well of 0-5-1 mg/ml p-nitrophenyl phosphate substrate in substrate buffer
19. Read the plate after 1 hour and or overnight

10. Positive and negative controls

For every ELISA test there are positive and negative controls which must be from the same genotype (s) as the samples. These are used to determine if the samples are infected. Two positive control samples well derived from plant infected with the virus to be diagnosed should be included in every test. Samples material used for negative control must come from plant that has tested negative for virus infection (KPL Technical Guide on line 1999/2000 edition; Jackie Hughes *et al* 2004).

11. ELISA plate layout

Determination of plate layout varies with the test to be carried out. New clean ELISA plates should be used for new test to avoid contamination. To avoid edge effect due to inconsistency of the results to be obtained, the outside wells should not be used for any test. Positive control wells are advised to be put at the top left hand corner while the negative control wells are put at the bottom right hand corner (KPL Technical Guide on line 1999/2000 edition; Jackie Hughes *et al* 2004). The remaining wells then serves as test sample wells using two wells per sample test. Non water soluble marker pens should be used to demarcate various test sample areas (Jackie Hughes *et al* (2004).

12. ELISA result interpretation

There are two basic type of ELISA reader. One reads the entire plate at once while the other reads individual well if correctly used. Plate's bottom to be read must be clean and dry and result read at room temperature. Contact the user's manual for the ELISA reader for further assistance. ELISA result is read using nanometer reading set at *A405 infection* ($A_{405\ inf}$) no matter the type of ELISA reader used (Jackie Hughes *et al* (2004). A sample test is considered positive for the virus if its ELISA reading doubles that of the negative control (KPL Technical Guide on line 1999/2000 edition). In some cases the sample test is considered virus positive if the ELISA reading is1.5 times the means of the negative controls (Jackie Hughes *et al* (2004);

13. Polymerase Chain Reaction (PCR)

This is a method for nucleic acid amplification *in-vitro*. The product of the polymerase chain reaction is been used by PCR for identification. It is highly sensitive; apart from identifying the DNA it also amplifies the target nucleic acid sequence (Dellaporta *et al.* 1983). It uses multiple cycles of template denaturation, primer annealing and primer elongation to amplify DNA sequence (Dellaporta *et al.* 1983; Jackie Hughes *et al* 2004). Each step occurring at specific temperature for specified time period.

Components of PCR as described by Dellaporta *et al.* (1983) and Jackie Hughes *et al* (2004)

Template: Nucleic acid of infected plant or virus DNA. RNA viruses are converted to cDNA before amplification.

Primers: Sequences of short fragment of oligonucleotides (single stranded DNA) complementary to the sequences at the end of target sequences to be amplified. Forward and reverse primers are required in this reaction.

dNTPs: Nucleotides required for the extension of the newly synthesized DNA strand. dATP, dCTP, dGTP, dTTP (the four neucleotides) are included in the mixture

Enzyme: A thermostable (heat resistant) enzyme is required for polymerization due that the polymerase reaction undergoes denaturation of template at high temperature. Taq polymerase is the thermostable polymerase enzyme used frequently.

13.1 Reaction buffer and magnesium chloride

The magnesium ion concentration affects among others, enzyme activity, primer annealing and denaturation (Jackie Hughes *et al* 2004).

PCR reaction is carried out in a thermo cycler that has been programmed to cycle between high and low temperatures within a specified period of time. This involves 3 main steps as described by Jackie Hughes *et al* (2004).

1. Template DNA denaturation
2. Annealing of primers
3. Extension of DNA strand

Two new DNA strands as explained by Jackie Hughes *et al* (2004) are formed at the end of the first cycle totaling four strands of DNA template which serves as templates for the second cycle. In the second cycle, the new DNA elongates as the primers binds to the templates. A total of eight strands would have been synthesized at the end of the second cycle. The DNA increases at exponential rate with each cycle as the PCR continues until set number of cycles has been reached. Ethidium bromide stained gel is used to visualize the final product (Dellaporta *et al.* 1983; Jackie Hughes *et al* 2004).

PCR Reaction mixture as described by Dellaporta *et al.* (1983) and Jackie Hughes *et al* (2004)

To detect individual viruses, specific primers are to be used.

Reagent	**Stock concentration**	**Working concentration**
Buffer	10x	1x
MgCl	25 mM	1.5 mM
dNTPs	20 mM	
Primer 1		10-100 pmole
Primer 2		10-100 pmole
Taq polymerase	5 units/ µl	0.8-2.5 units
DNA		1-10 ng

13.2 Reverse Transcriptase PCR (RT-PCR)

Viruses with RNA are amplified with reverse transcriptase as their nucleic acid in PCR. DNA is used as template for Taq polymerase; therefore the virus will have to convert its RNA to cDNA before the polymerase reaction. Short cDNA are formed due to cleavages caused in the RNA due to the contaminating RNase. One-tube reaction or two-tube reactions can be used to carry out RT-PCR (Dellaporta *et al.* 1983; Jackie Hughes *et al* 2004).

13.3 Two-tube RT-PCR

RNA extracted from the virus as template or total nucleic acid extracted from the infected plant is used to synthesize cDNA by reverse transcription. An aliquot of the reverse transcription reaction is used in the PCR. Usually, not more than 1/5 of the total PCR mixture should derived from the reverse transcription reaction (Jackie Hughes *et al* 2004).

13.4 One-tube RT-PCR

This is where the same buffer is used to carry out the reverse-transcription reaction and PCR so the two reactions can not be separately optimized. Before adding the mixture, the RNA need to be denatured at 70-75°C for 5 min so that there can be good synthesis of cDNA which is immediately followed with a PCR cycling programme (Jackie Hughes *et al* 2004). The thermocycler can accommodate both programmes at the same time as one programme (Jackie Hughes *et al* 2004).

13.5 Immunocapture PCR

Along with the PCR the virus particle could be trapped using the antiserums. This reaction could be carried out in a single tube. This method is good for viruses having low concentration in the plant or viruses having their genome integrated into host plant genome (Dellaporta *et al.* 1983; Jackie Hughes *et al* 2004).

13.6 Immunocapture reverse transcription PCR

In this test RNA is used as the template which makes it differs from immuno-capture PCR which make it very efficient in detecting RNA in viruses from plant that could have affected the enzymes in the reverse transcription reaction or the PCR through some inhibitory compounds that it contains (Jackie Hughes *et al* 2004). A single tube can be used to carry out immuno-capture, reverse transcription and the PCR and the different reactions could be carried out separately.

An example of a typical IC-RT-PCR as described by Jackie Hughes *et al* (2004).

1. Coat tubes with polyclonal antibodies diluted in coating buffer (200µl)
2. Incubate at 37^{0}C for 2-3 hours
3. Wash tubes with PBS-Tween
4. Add 200µl of sample ground in (ELISA) sample buffer
5. Incubate overnight at 4^{0}C or 2-3 hr at 37^{0}C
6. Wash two times with PBS-Tween
7. Add RT-PCR mix and subject to thermal cycling consisting of one cycle of RT

RT-PCR Mix

10x PCR buffer	1x
MgCl	2.0 mM
dNTPs mix	0.5 mM
Primers	10 pmole each
Taq DNA polymerase	2.5 units
Reverse Trancriptase	200 units
RNase free water	_
Total volume	25-50 µl

Cycling condition should consist of an initial one cycle for the reverse transcription linked to the PCR cycle.

14. Extraction of DNA for PCR

The DNA extraction procedure as developed by Jackie Hughes *et al* (2004).

1. Grind about 50mg of young infected plant material in 500 µl of extraction buffer
2. Pour sap into a new and sterilized Eppendorf tube.
3. Add 33ul of 20% sodium dodecyl sulphate (sds)
4. Vortex briefly and incubate in water bath at 65^{0}C for 10 min
5. Bring to room temperature and add 160ul of 5M potassium acetate
6. Vortex and centrifuge at 10,000 g for 10 min
7. Remove the supernatant (about 400 µl) into another Eppendorf tube
8. Add 200 µl of cold iso-propanol
9. Mix gently and keep on ice or at 4^{0}C for 15-20 min
10. Centrifuge at 10,000 g for 10 min to sediment the DNA
11. Decant the supernatant gently and ensure that the pellet is not disturbed
12. Add 500 µl of 70% ethanol to the pellet (this is to wash it) and centrifuge at 10,000g for 5-10 min.

13. Decant the ethanol and air-dry the DNA (at room temp) until no trace of alcohol can be seen in ht tube.

The DNA is re-suspended in 950 µl TE or sterile distilled water) and stored in the freeze as stock solution. The DNA is usually diluted $1x10^5$ times for PCR, but it will be better do a dilution curve to determine the best dilution for amplification.

Extraction buffer
100 mM (pH 8.0)
8.5 mM EDTA
500 mM NaCl
10 mM β-mercaptoethanol (added just before use)

TE buffer
10 mM Tris
1 mM EDTA

Extraction of total nucleic acids for RT-PCR (Method A) as described by Jackie Hughes *et al* (2004)

1. Grind 50-100 mg of young leaf sample in 500 µl of extraction buffer using cooled sterilized pestle and mortar.
2. Add proteinase K and SDS to a final concentration of 50 mg/ml and 0.1% respectively.
3. Incubate the mixture at 37⁰C for 5 min
4. Add 500 µl of phenol and vortex for a few seconds.
5. Centrifuge at 5,000g for 5 min.
6. Remove the aqueous phase into another Eppendorf tube
7. Add 35 µl of chloroform and vortex briefly
8. Remove the aqueous phase and repeat the chloroform extraction..
9. Remove the aqueous phase into another Eppendorf tube and add 1/10 volume of 3 M sodium acetate and twice the volume of colf ethanol and precipitate nucleic acid overnight at -20⁰C.
10. Spin at 10,000g for 15 min and pour off the ethanol.
11. Wash nucleic acid with 70% ethanol.
12. Dry nucleic acid at room temperature.
13. Re-suspend nucleic acid in 20 µl of sterile distilled water.

14.1 Extraction buffer

50 mM Tris-HCl pH 8.0
10 mM EDTA
1 mM DTT
50 mM NaCl

Extraction of total nucleic acid for PCR (Method B) as described by Jackie Hughes *et al* (2004).

1. Grind 50-100 mg leaf sample in liquid nitrogen.
2. Add 600 µl of CTAB buffer and mix thoroughly.
3. Incubate at 55⁰ C for 15-30 min
4. Shake mixture with 300 µl of choroform; isomyl alcohol (24:1)

5. Centrifuge at 10,000g for 5 min.
6. Remove the aqueous phase into a fresh Eppendorf tube and add tenth volume of 7.5-ammonium acetate or 3 M sodium acetate.
7. Add equal volume of iso-propanol and keep for 15 min at 4^0C
8. Centrifuge at 10,000 g for 10 min and wash the pellet with 70% ethanol
9. Dry total nucleic acid at room temperature.

14.2 CTAB buffer

Cetyltrimethyl ammonium bromide	2% (w/v)
NaCl	1.4 M
Tris-HCl (pH 8.0)	0.1M
β-mercaptoethanol	0.5%

15. Electrophoresis of nucleic acids

Nucleic acids can be size fractionated in agarose or polyacrtlamide gels (Dellaporta *et al.* 1983). Agarose gels are frequently used because it is easy to prepare and safer compared to polyacrylamide (Dellaporta *et al.* 1983). The nucleic acid is stained with ethidium bromide that can be incorporated in the gel during preparation or stained after electrophoresis. Nucleic acids migrate towards the positive pole in an electric field in an appropriate buffer (Dellaporta *et al.* 1983; Jackie Hughes *et al* 2004).

15.1 Electrophoresis and gel loading buffer

Tris acetate buffer (TAE) and Tris-orate buffer are the commonly used electrophoresis buffer

Preparation of an Agarose Gel as described by Jackie Hughes *et al* (2004)

1. Seal the ends of the plastic tray supplied with the electrophoresis apparatus with tape.
2. Prepare sufficient electrophoresis buffer to fill the tank and to prepare the gel, measure the quantity of agarose required into an Erlenmeyer flask or glass bottle with a loose-fitting cap and add the buffer to the agarose to give the required concentration of gel (usually 1%w/v is used for most analyses.
3. Heat the agarose suspension in a microwave oven or a heater until it boils and dissolves
4. Cool solution to 60^0C and if desired add anthodium bromide (from a stock solution of 10 mg/ml in water) to a final concentration of 0.5 μg/'ml and mix thoroughly.
5. Position the comb in the tank. If the comb is too close to the plate, there is a risk that the base of the well may tear when the comb is withdrawn, allowing the sample to leak between the gel and the plate.
6. Pour the agarose into the prepared tray and allow to set at room temperature.
7. After the gel is completely set (30-45 min) carefully remove the comb and tape and mount the gel in the electrophoresis tank.
8. Add enough electrophoresis buffers to cover the gel to a depth of about 1mm.
9. Mix the sample DNA with the desired gel-loading buffer and slowly load the mixture into the slots of the submerged gel using a disposable micropipette.

10. Attach electrical leads to the tank so that the DNA will migrate toward the anode (usually the red lead). Apply a voltage 1-5 V/cm to the gel. Run the gel until the bromophenol blue has migrated an appropriate distance from the gel.
11. Turn off the electric current and remove the leads. If ethidium bromide is present in the gel, examine the gel by ultraviolet light.

If the anthodium bromide was not added to the gel, the gel must be stained by soaking in a solution containing ethidium bromide (0.5 μg/ml) for about 30-45 min.

16. References

Dellaporta S.L., Wood J. and Hicks J.B. 1983. A plant DNA mini-preparation Version II. *Plant Molecular Biology Reporter 1*: 19-21

Fajinmi AA. 2006. The incidence, spread and possible control strategies of *Pepper veinal Mottle Potyvirus* (PVMV) disease on pepper (*Capsicum annuum*. L.) in Nigeria. *PhD thesis*, University of Ibadan, Oyo State, Nigeria.

Fajinmi, A. A. (2011) 'Agro-ecological incidence and severity of *Pepper veinal mottle virus*, genus *Potyvirus*, family *Potyviridae*, on cultivated pepper (*Capsicum annuum* L.) in Nigeria', *Archives of Phytopathology and Plant Protection*, 44: 4, 307 – 319

KPL Technical Guide for ELISA Protocols (on line 1999/2000 edition) KPL, Inc* 800-638-3167 * 301-948-7755 * www.kpl.com

Jackie Hughes, Sam Offei, Blake Rollenfitch. 2004. Plant viruses in Sub-Saharan Africa. A Practical Laboratory Manual. International Institute of Tropical Agriculture, Ibadan, Nigeria. 2004.

6

Serology Applied to Plant Virology

J. Albersio A. Lima[1], Aline Kelly Q. Nascimento[1],
Paula Radaelli[1] and Dan E. Purcifull[2]
[1]*Federal University of Ceará,*
Laboratory of Plant Virology,
Fortaleza, CE,
[2]*Gainesville, FL,*
[1]*Brazil*
[2]*USA*

1. Introduction

Virus infections affect seriously the quality and quantity of agricultural products around the world, especially in less developed countries. For this reason, the development and the adaptation of efficient and rapid techniques for diagnosis and control of plant viruses constitute an imperative and relevant necessity. Attempting to control plant diseases including those caused by viruses without sufficient information about their causal agents, their dissemination and surviving properties, usually results in inadequate control and many times, in a total failure. So, any attempt to establish a control program for a plant disease must be, always, preceded by a correct and precise laboratory diagnosis.

Several methods can be used for arriving at a correct and definitive diagnosis of plant disease caused by virus and at the beginning of the study of plant virology, the symptoms represented important characteristics for plant virus identification and characterization (Almeida & Lima, 2001; Astier et al., 2007; Mulholland, 2009; Naidu & Hughes, 2001; Purcifull et al., 2001). Nevertheless, it is often impossible to diagnose plant virus infections merely by observing host symptoms because symptoms caused by viruses vary according to the plant variety involved, the environmental conditions, the strain of the virus, the fact that sometimes different viruses can cause similar symptoms in the same plant species and sometimes the disease could result from the synergistic effect of infection caused by two different viruses. Additionally, symptoms may be very slight and inconclusive, or infected plants may be symptomless. However, bioassay through the use of a series of indicator plants remains an indispensable tool for detection and identification of plant viruses and the original symptoms are still of great importance for plant virus denomination (Astier et al., 2007; Lima et al., 2005; Mulholland, 2009).

Over the last few decades, laboratory-based methods have been developed and are now being used routinely in many laboratories for accurate diagnosis of diseases caused by plant viruses. These techniques involve physical, biological, cytological, serological, and molecular properties of viruses. Numerous laboratory methods have been developed and adapted for virus diagnosis, but serology is one of the most specific and easiest methods to obtain a rapid and precise identification (Astier et al., 2007; Koenig et al., 2008; Lima et al., 2005; Naidu & Hughes, 2001; Purcifull et al., 2001). Serological assays have been developed and used successfully for many years for plant virus detection. Plant Disease is a journal that publishes papers that deal significantly with diagnosis and control of plant virus diseases. Of 164 papers published on plant viruses in 22 issues of this journal during 2010-2011, the authors of 115 papers (70%) utilized serology for virus diagnosis or detection. Enzyme-linked immunosorbent assay (ELISA) methods were used extensively (the authors of 105 papers utilized ELISA). Other serological techniques that were used included tissue blot immunoassays, immunoelectron microscopy (trapping and decoration), Western blots, dot blots, lateral flow rapid tests, immunocapture PCR, and double diffusion tests. Serological tests may be decisive in the final identification of an unknown virus and may be important in studying the relationship between virus species and strains. The great value of serological methods for plant virus identification is based on the specific reaction between the viral antigens and their specific antibodies. An antigen is a molecule that when injected into a vertebrate animal (usually a mammal or a bird), it can trigger an immune response in the animal which results in production of specific antibodies that can combine with the foreign antigen (Astier et al., 2007; Lima et al., 2005; Naidu & Hughes, 2001; Purcifull et al., 2001). Virus particles themselves and their proteins have several antigenic determinants (epitopes) which vary in their amino acid sequence and have the properties of inducing the production of specific antibodies. The virus particles, their coat proteins and the other types of virus induced proteins including those found in inclusion bodies can function as antigens (Astier et al., 2007; Hiebert, et al., 1984; Lima et al., 2005; Naidu & Hughes, 2001; Purcifull et al., 2001).

Antibodies are also proteins of the immunoglobulin group (Ig) produced against specific antigenic determinants and are present in the animal blood. The immunoglobulin G (IgG) is the most common type of Ig produced and, consequently most commonly involved in the serological tests for plant virus identification. This type of antibody is composed of four linked polypeptides with Y-shape of approximately 150 Kd, with two identical heavy chains and two identical light chains of polypeptides (Figure 1). The IgG has two identical combining sites specific for antigenic determinants called paratopes in the NH_2 terminal regions of the heave and light chains. These two identical combining sites have highly variable amino acid sequence, which permit the production of specific IgGs for the different virus epitopes. The C-terminal regions of the heavy chains are linked together by sulfur bridges to produce the Fc fraction of the antibody (Figure 1) which links specifically with protein A or cell membranes (Almeida, 2001; Purcifull et al., 2001).

Generally the methods that involve the antigen antibody reactions *in vitro* are simple and do not require sophisticated and expensive apparatus. The most serious limitation to using serology for plant virus identification and detection is the difficulty in producing a good virus specific antiserum. Most antisera used for plant virus identification and detection are usually prepared by immunizing mammals or birds with purified plant virus or their different types of proteins. However several other methods have been used to produce very specific antibodies, including monoclonal antibody (Mab) which consists of a single type of antibody that reacts with only one specific epitope of a virus protein. The production of Mab consists of a series of steps, including mouse immunization, collection of antibody producing cells, fusion with myeloma cells to produce a *hybridoma*, screening and selection process of *hybridoma* specific for the desired virus epitope. The *hybridoma* cells obtained can be stored in a freezer and used to produce the same monoclonal antibody according to necessity (Cancino et al., 1995; Purcifull et al. 2001). Monoclonal antibodies have been used, for instance, to study antigenic differences and relationships among virus strains. Examples include studies of the relationships among strains of potyviruses that infect cucurbits (Baker et al., 1991; Desbiez et al., 2007)

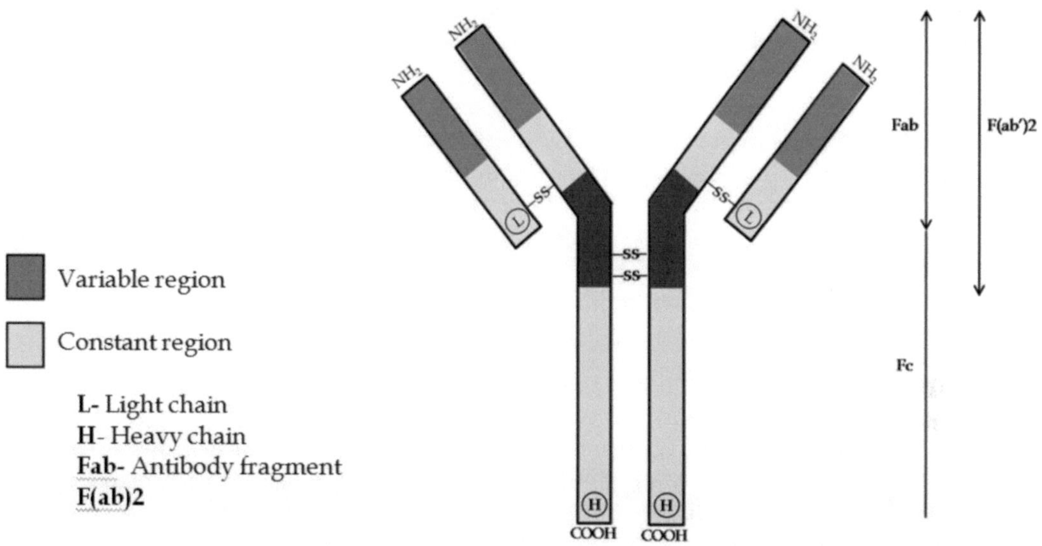

Fig. 1. Diagrammatic representation of the structure of an immunoglobulin G (IgG) molecule. Fab, F(ab)2, and Fc represent fragments obtained by enzyme cleavage of IgG.

Considering the importance of serology for diagnosing and surveying plant virus diseases, a program of polyclonal antiserum production for plant viruses was established at the Plant Virus Laboratory from the Federal University of Ceará (PVLab/UFC) in Northeastern Brazil, since the beginning of 1978. The serological plant virus survey program has been essential for establishing control programs such as roguing of virus infected plants in papaya (*Carica papaya* L.) orchards, indexing for production of virus free nurseries of banana (*Musa* spp.), melon (*Cucumis melo* L.) and watermelon [*Citrullus lanatus* (Thumb.) Matsum. & Nakai Mansf.], for production of virus-free seeds of cowpea [*Vigna unguiculata* (L.) Walp. subsp. *unguiculata*] and for selecting sources of virus resistance in cowpea, melon and watermelon. Polyclonal antisera specific for several virus species and strains that infect tropical crops have been produced at the PVLab/UFC (Table 1).

Banana plantation is expanding in the Northeast of Brazil but surveys using enzyme-linked immunosorbent assay (ELISA) and polymerase chain reaction (PCR) had shown that its productivity is still affected by *Cucumber mosaic virus* (CMV) family *Bromoviridae* genus *Cucumovirus* and *Banana streak virus* (BSV) family *Badnaviridae* genus *Caulimovirus* (Nascimento et al., 2011).

More than 20 virus species were found naturally infecting different cucurbit species, but only five species were serologically detected and isolated in Northeastern Brazil, including those that belong to the following families and genera: family *Bromoviridae* genus *Cucumovirus*: *Cucumber mosaic virus* (CMV); family *Comoviridae* genus *Comovirus*: *Squash mosaic virus* (SQMV) and family *Potyviridae* genus *Potyvirus*: *Papaya ringspot virus*, type

Watermelon (PRSV-W); *Watermelon mosaic virus* (WMV) and *Zucchini yellow mosaic virus* (ZYMV) (Lima & Amaral, 1985; Moura et al., 2001; Oliveira et al., 2000; 2002).

Several factors affect papaya productivity in Northeastern Brazil, mainly the infectious diseases caused by viruses, which have been responsible for great losses in the crop throughout the country (Barbosa & Paguio, 1982; Lima & Gomes, 1975; Lima et al., 2001; Nascimento et al., 2010; Ventura, 2004). The most important viruses that infect papaya in Northeastern Brazil are *Papaya ringspot virus* (PRSV), family *Potyviridae*, genus *Potyvirus* (Lima & Gomes, 1975); *Papaya lethal yellowing virus* (PLYV), possible family *Sobemoviridae*, genus *Sobemovirus* (Nascimento et al., 2010) and *Papaya meleira virus* (PMeV), which is still being characterized to be classified taxonomically by the ICTV (Marciel-Zambolim et al., 2003). Among the major virus diseases of passion fruit is the woodiness caused by *Passion fruit woodiness virus* (PWV) and *Cowpea aphid borne mosaic virus* (CABMV), both from the family *Potyviridae*, genus *Potyvirus*. These viruses cause great damage to the plant, inducing mottle, mosaic in young leaves, reduction of apical internodes, woodiness, deformation and reduction of fruit size (Bezerra et al., 1995).

Cowpea that is part of the traditional agricultural system of the semi-arid region of Brazil is largely infected with several virus species (Lima et al., 2005) including those from the following families and genera (Lima et al., 2005): family *Comoviridae* genus *Comovirus*: *Cowpea severe mosaic virus* (CPSMV); family *Potyviridae* genus *Potyvirus*: *Cowpea aphid-borne mosaic virus* (CABMV); family *Bromoviridae* genus *Cucumovirus*: *Cucumber mosaic virus* (CMV) and family *Gemniviridae* the genus *Begomovirus*: *Cowpea golden mosaic virus* (CGMV) (Florindo & Lima, 1991; Lima et al., 1979; 1991; 1993).

2. Polyclonal antiserum production

Most plant viruses are good and effective antigens which when artificially injected into a suitable vertebrate animal stimulate the production of specific antibodies that can be used in various serological tests. The rabbits are the most common animal choice in polyclonal antiserum production since they are easily housed and adapt well to being handled, but other animals such as mice, goats and chickens can be used. Nevertheless, the serious limitation in using serology for plant virus identification is the difficulty in producing a high titer virus specific antiserum. Through necessity, specific plant virus antisera have been produced in many different Plant Virus Research Laboratories throughout the world. Often, these collections have served as a major source of antisera for commercial companies that sell plant virus antisera and diagnosis services on an international basis. The PVLab/UFC in the State of Ceará, Brazil has been given an important collaboration in the production of antisera for tropical plant viruses (Table 1) and in the development and adaptation of serological techniques for plant virus identification since the 1970-decade (Lima & Amaral, 1985; Lima & Nelson, 1977; Lima et al., 1993; 1994; 2001; 2005; Nascimento et al., 2010; Oliveira et al., 2000; 2002). However, some virus isolates already identified at family and genus levels have been maintained in greenhouses for purification and subsequently antiserum production.

The production of antiserum for some plant viruses is, mainly, limited by the difficulty in purifying such viruses free from plant protein contaminants and in appropriate concentration to be used as antigen. Several other methods have been developed for plant

Crop/Virus specie/ Strain	Quantity of Antiserum (ml)	Number of samples in ELISA (1:2,000)*
Lettuce: *Lactuca sativa* L.		
Lettuce mosaic virus (LMV)	122	1,220,000
Curcubitaceae		
Cucumber mosaic virus (CMV)	422	4,220,000
Papaya ringspot virus - Watermelon (PRSV-W)	210	2,100,000
Squash mosaic virus (SQMV)	380	3,800,000
Watermelon mosaic virus (WMV)	191	1,910,000
Zucchini yellow mosaic virus (ZYMV)	62	620,000
Leguminosae		
Bean common mosaic virus (BCMV)	112	1,120,000
Blackeye cowpea mosaic virus (BlCMV)	90	900,000
Cowpea aphid-borne mosaic virus (CABMV)	429	4,290,000
Soybean mosaic virus (SoyMV)	85	850,000
Cowpea severe mosaic virus (CPSMV)		
$CPSMV_{CE}$	530	5,300,000
$CPSMV_{MC}$	311	3,110,000
$CPSMV_{CROT}$	320	3,200,000
$CPSMV_{AL}$	208	2,080,000
$CPSMV_{PB}$	125	1,250,000
Papaya: *Carica papaya* L.		
Papaya yellow mosaic virus (PLYV)	285	2,850,000
Papaya ringspot virus - Watermelon (PRSV-W)	210	2,100,000
Passionfruit: *Passiflora edulis* Sims.		
Cucumber mosaic virus (CMV)	422	4,220,000
Passion fruit woodiness virus (PWV)	42	420,000

Table 1. Polyclonal antisera specific for plant virus species that infect tropical crops produced in the Plant Virus Laboratory from the Federal University of Ceará (PVLab/UFC). * Number of samples that could be tested with available antiserum diluted 1:2,000 using 100 µl per well and replication of each sample.

virus antigen production, including the transformation of bacterial cells with the virus coat protein gene. This chapter will describe the most commonly used method to produce polyclonal antibodies specific for plant virus detection and identification. The process describes the production of polyclonal antibodies by rabbit immunization with purified virus preparations (Figure 2). Although not very specific for virus species/strains discrimination, the polyclonal antiserum is very useful and practical for virus surveys and indexing.

Several routes have been used to immunize rabbits with plant viruses, including intravenous, intramuscular and through the foot pad. The protocols of rabbit immunization vary greatly, but the following general immunization procedure has given satisfactory results for preparation of good titter plant virus antiserum. A rabbit is immunized with purified virus preparation by three weekly injections, using in each immunization an aliquot of 500 µl from the purified virus preparation (0.5-1.0 mg/ml) emulsified with equal volume of Freund incomplete adjuvant. The emulsified virus preparation is injected into the thigh

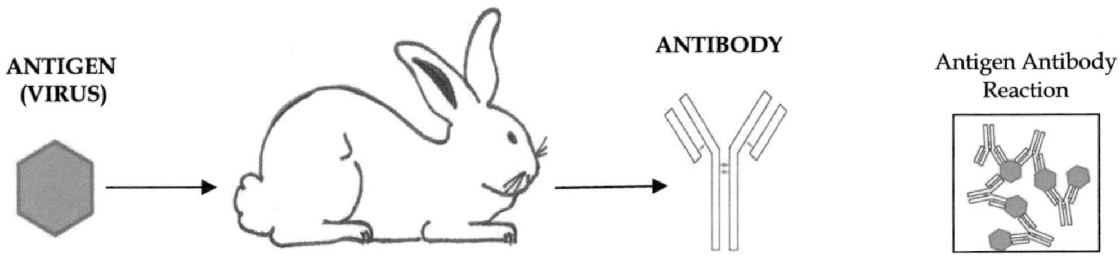

Fig. 2. Principle of polyclonal antiserum production specific for plant virus.

muscle of each hind leg or into the foot pad of the animal, and 15 days after the last injection the rabbit could be bled for antiserum production. Blood samples of 10 to up 50 ml are taken by nicking the marginal ear vein of the animal and collecting in glass centrifuge tubes. The tubes with the blood samples are maintained in a water bath at 37 °C for one hour and then centrifuged at 4,000 g for 10 min. The serum should be drained from the clots in conical-bottom tubes and centrifuged at 10,000 g for 15 min (Almeida & Lima, 2001; Purcifull & Batchelor, 1977). The clear supernatant serum from the second centrifugation is collected, evaluated by indirect ELISA and/or Ouchterlony double-diffusion tests (Almeida & Lima, 2001; Ouchterlony, 1962; Purcifull & Batchelor, 1977) and stored at -20 °C.

Antisera for some plant viruses were also obtained by oral immunization of rabbit or mouse with purified viruses or even with concentrated leaf extracts of infected plants (Florindo & Lima, 1991). Antiserum specific for CPSMV, SQMV and PLYV were obtained by immunizing rabbits with partially purified preparations or with foliar extracts of infected plants prepared in 0.15 M NaCl solution, in a proportion of 1:1 (w/v), clarified by centrifugation at 10,000 g for 10 min, using daily doses, for a period of seven days (Rabelo Filho et al., 2005).

3. Serological methods

Numerous serological techniques have been developed for identification and characterization of plant viruses and the advent of the enzyme-linked immunosorbent assay (ELISA) has facilitated the use of serology for virus identification in large scale (Astier et al., 2007; Hampton et al., 1990; Lima et al., 2005; Naidu & Hughes, 2001; Nascimento et al., 2010; Purcifull et al., 2001; Van Regenmortel, 1982; Van Regenmortel & Dubs, 1993). All the serological techniques for virus identifications are based on the virus coat protein properties. The serological methods can be subdivided into two broader categories involving liquid and solid phase methods. The liquid phase methods can be represented by the double immune diffusion techniques in which the antigen and the antibodies react in agar media producing visible precipitates. In the solid phase methods, one of the reagents, usually the antibody, is trapped on a solid surface that could be nitrocellulose membrane, a microtitre plate, polystyrene or polyvinyl chloride plates. In this case the antigen-antibody reaction is detected by a labeled antibody as in the ELISA and its variations. In addition the virus particles are detected by direct visualization as with serologically specific electron microscopy (SSEM). An overview of SSEM, double immune diffusion technique, ELISA and its different variations will be provided in the following sections, including some illustrations, but detailed descriptions can be found in Van Regenmortel (1982), Hampton et al. (1990), Torrance (1992), Van Regenmortel & Dubs (1993), Purcifull et al. (2001) and Naidu & Hughes (2001).

3.1 Enzyme-Linked Immunosorbent Assay (ELISA)

ELISA is a very specific and sensitive serological technique introduced to the study and identification of plant viruses in the 1970s (Clark & Adams, 1977; Voller et al., 1976). This technique is able to detect virus particles in very low concentrations and can be used with viruses of different particle morphology. Because of its adaptability, high sensitivity, and economy in the use of reagents, ELISA is used in a wide range of situations, especially for indexing a large number of samples in a relatively short period of time. The ELISA technique is based on the basic principle in which the virus antigens are recognized by their specific antibodies (IgG) in association with colorimetric properties. The ELISA method is commonly accomplished in a 96-well polystyrene plate by adding the antigens and antibodies into the wells in an established sequence, involving several stages (Figure 3 A, B). In the final stage, the positive reactions are detected when a colorless substrate, usually p-nitrophenyl phosphate, undergoes a chemical change resulting in a yellow colored product as the result of exposure to the enzyme alkaline phosphate linked to the antibody. The degree of color change indicates the degree of reactivity that is read by an ELISA plate reader apparatus. It is always recommended to include a homologous antigen for the specific virus antibody and extracts from healthy plants to compare the absorption readings and to obtain a correct interpretation of the results. Differently from some other serological tests, the principle of ELISA techniques consists of detecting the antigen-antibody interactions by enzyme induced color reaction rather than by observing their precipitation. Although different variations of this serological technique have been developed, the direct and the indirect ELISA (Figure 3) are the most frequently used methods for diagnosis of plant virus diseases (Almeida & Lima, 2001; Clark & Bar-Joseph 1984; Cooper & Edwards 1986; Van Regenmortel & Dubs 1993). It is always recommended to include a homologous antigen (positive control) for the specific virus antibody and extracts from healthy plants (negative control) to compare the absorption readings and to obtain a correct interpretation of the results

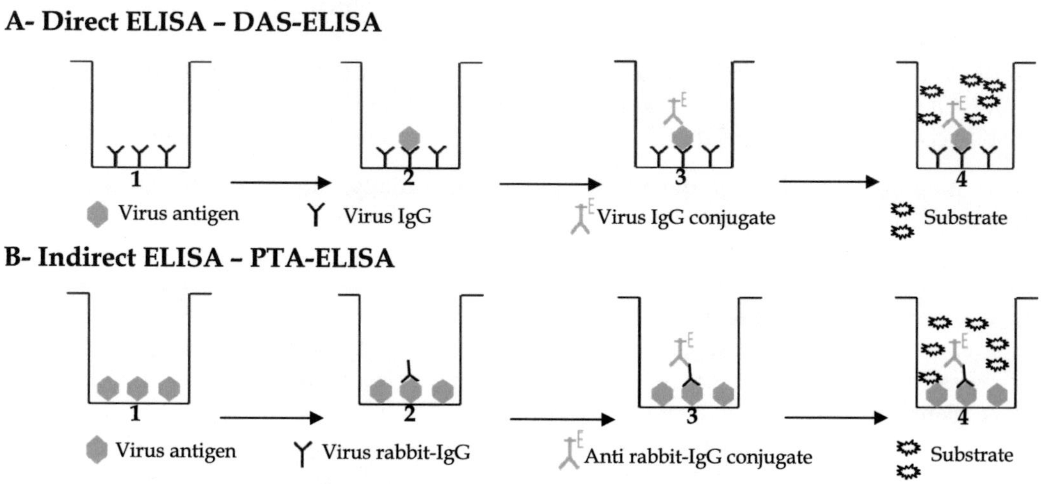

Fig. 3. Diagrammatic drawings of the most frequently used methods for detection of plant viruses: A- Direct ELISA and B- Indirect ELISA.

3.1.1 Direct ELISA

The direct ELISA (Figure 3A), also called double antibody sandwich (DAS-ELISA), is highly strain-specific and requires each detecting antibody to be conjugated to an enzyme. Typically, the enzyme is alkaline phosphatase. The first step in the test is the adsorption of virus-specific antibodies to the wells of ELISA plates. Unbound antibody is removed by washing, and the samples to be tested for virus antigen are added. Controls include extracts from known infected plants (positive control), and extracts from healthy plants (negative control). After incubation and washing, the enzyme-antibody conjugate is added. If virus attached to the coating antibody is present, the enzyme-antibody conjugate will combine with the virus. Plates are washed, and the colorless substrate (p-nitrophenylphosphate) is added. Positive wells will show a yellow reaction, due to the action of the conjugated enzyme (alkaline phosphatase) on the substrate. Negative wells will remain colorless. The colorimetric changes are measured in an ELISA reader, using a filter for 405 nm wave length. The washing procedures can be accomplished by the use of a plate washing apparatus, according to a programmed schedule. The quality of the antiserum is critical in achieving certain objectives, but a good, broad spectrum polyclonal antiserum will give satisfactory results in most virus indexing programs. On the other hand, monoclonal antibodies could be useful for identification and characterization of specific plant virus strains.

3.1.2 Indirect ELISA

Although the direct ELISA technique has high sensitivity and specificity, a method called indirect ELISA or plate-trapped antigen (PTA- ELISA) was developed to avoid the inconveniences and the difficulties of conjugating the enzyme with the IgG specific for each virus species to be used in the second layer of antibodies in direct ELISA. For this reason, the indirect ELISA or PTA-ELISA requires antibodies produced in two different animal species and the virus particles are trapped in the wells of the ELISA plate. The indirect ELISA also requires the use of a universal IgG enzyme conjugate which can be used with the antibodies of all virus species. The so called universal conjugate is composed of an IgG produced against the IgGs from the animal in which virus antibodies are raised linked to the enzyme alkaline phosphate. If the virus antibodies are produced in rabbits (e.g.), an anti-rabbit IgGs are produced in a second animal species such as goats or mice. So, the detecting antibody conjugate binds specifically to the primary virus specific antibody (Figure 3B).

In this method, the wells of the ELISA plate are, initially, covered with extracts from infected and healthy plant samples prepared in the proportion of 1:10 in carbonate buffer, pH 9.6. Following that, the virus particles are covered with a layer of virus specific antibodies produced in a rabbit, for example. The complex antigen-antibodies are covered with a universal conjugate that could be an anti-rabbit IgG produced in goats or mice linked to the enzyme alkaline phosphate. The linked anti-IgG-enzyme that react with the virus antibodies (IgG) which had reacted with the virus particles adsorbed to the bottom of the ELISA plate wells will be detected by colorimetric changes of a specific substrate that is added into the wells. Considering that a single universal antibody-conjugate can be used for detection of a wide range of plant viruses, the indirect ELISA technique is more economical, practical and suitable for virus detection in disease diagnosis and quarantine programs. For this reason, this ELISA technique is described in more detail in this chapter. Nevertheless, this method has certain disadvantages such as competition between plant sap and virus particles for sites on the plate wells and, consequently, high background reactions. Although the indirect ELISA technique is not very specific for plant virus strain identification, it can be used for virus species differentiation by antiserum cross absorption. Using indirect ELISA, Oliveira et al. (2000) demonstrated that an isolate of *Papaya ringspot virus* type watermelon (PRSV-W) genus *Potyvirus* is serologically different from *Watermelon mosaic virus* (WMV) and *Zucchini yellow mosaic virus* (ZYMV) also from the genus *Potyvirus* while isolates of WMV and ZYMV showed strong relationship with some differences that could be detected by reciprocal cross absorption with homologous and heterologous polyclonal antisera specific for WMV and ZYMV in indirect ELISA (Figure 4).

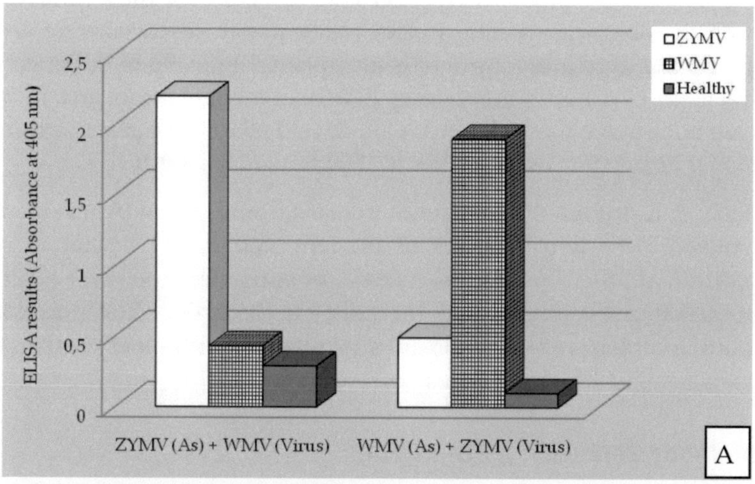

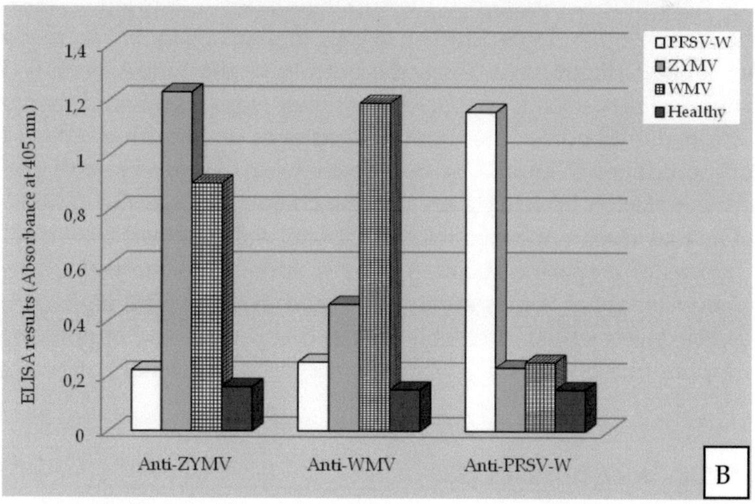

Fig. 4. Results of indirect ELISA showing serological relationship among *Papaya ringspot virus* type watermelon (PRSV-W), *Watermelon mosaic virus* (WMV) and *Zucchini yellow mosaic virus* (ZYMV), using polyclonal antisera. A) Reciprocal serological tests with antiserum for each virus species; B) Reciprocal indirect ELISA with polyclonal antisera for WMV and ZYMV absorbed with the heterologous virus species.

The complete indirect ELISA protocol consists of, initially, covering the plate wells with extracts from infected and healthy plant tissues prepared in the proportion of 1:10 in carbonate buffer, pH 9.6 and the plates are incubated at 37 ^{0}C for 1 h. The plates are washed three times with PBS Tween buffer and 100 µl of the virus polyclonal antiserum produced in rabbit previously absorbed by extracts from healthy plants, diluted to 2,000 to 6,000 are added into the wells. The plates are incubated again at 37 ^{0}C for 1 h, after which they are washed three times with PBS-Tween. After drying, 100 µl of anti-rabbit IgG produced in goat or mouse conjugated to alkaline phosphatase, diluted in the proportion of 1:2,000 to 1:6,000 in a buffer contain 2% of polyvinylpyrrolidone, 0.2% of albumin and 0.02% of sodium azide are added into the wells. The plates are incubated once more at 37 ^{0}C for 1 h and washed again three times with PBS-Tween. The washing procedures can be accomplished by the use of a washing ELISA plates apparatus, according to programmed schedules. Finally, 100 µl of a substrate of p-nitrophenyl phosphate in the concentration of 0.5 mg/ml dissolved in a buffer containing 12% of diethanolamine and 0.25% of sodium azide, pH 9.8 are added into the wells. After 20, 40 and 60 min the plates are analyzed in the ELISA plate reader apparatus, using a filter for 405 nm wave length.

For the polyclonal antiserum absorption with extracts from healthy plants one volume of the antiserum is mixed with two volumes of concentrated healthy plant extracts and the mixture is incubated at 37 ^{o}C for 3 h. The mixture of antiserum and plant healthy extracts is centrifuged at 10,000 g for 10 min and the pellet is discarded. The polyclonal absorbed antiserum should not interfere with the results by reacting with plant proteins from extracts for healthy plants in all ELISA procedures.

3.1.3 Triple Antibody Sandwich (TAS- ELISA)

Another widely used ELISA variation is the triple antibody sandwich (TAS- ELISA), which is similar to the direct ELISA (DAS- ELISA), except that an additional antibody produced in another animal is used (Figure 5A). First, the bottom of the ELISA plate wells are coated with a virus antibody produced in a species of animal (e.g., rabbit) and the virus antigen is linked in the trapped antibodies. The virus antigen is covered with a second layer of virus specific antibody produced in another animal species (e.g., mouse or goat) and the presence of this antibody is detected by adding an enzyme-conjugated specific antibody (e.g., rabbit anti-mouse IgG), that does not react with the plate well trapped antibody, followed by colorimetric changes of a specific substrate that is added into the wells. Considering that virus specific monoclonal antibodies are usually used in the second layer of antibodies this procedure is an effective method of combining the broad reactivity of polyclonal antibodies in the virus trapping phase with the specificities of the monoclonal antibodies (Purcifull et al., 2001).

3.1.4 Protein A-Sandwich (PAS- ELISA)

This ELISA variation is based on the property of protein A combining specifically with the Fc portion of the IgG. The protein A is obtained from the cell wall of *Staphylococcus aureus* and has a molecular weight of approximately 42 - 56 Kd (Almeida, 2001). This protein is very stable at a broad pH range and it is produced commercially, including a protein A-enzyme conjugate to be used in plant virology. It is prepared by direct dilution in pure

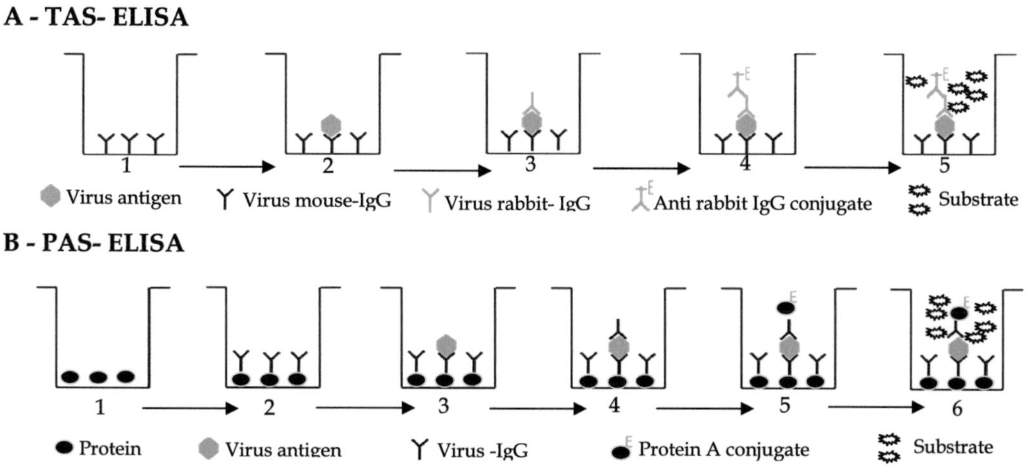

Fig. 5. Diagrammatic drawings of two ELISA variations for detection plant viruses: A) Triple antibody sandwich (TAS- ELISA) and B) Protein A-sandwich (PAS- ELISA).

water (1 mg/ml) and diluted in ELISA buffer to determine its adequate concentration for good results in PAS-ELISA. In the PAS-ELISA the antibody–virus–antibody layers which occur in the direct ELISA are sandwiched between two layers of protein A. The method consists of coating the bottom of the ELISA plate wells with a layer of protein A before the addition of the trapped virus antibody. Since the Fc region from the antibodies (IgG) has affinity to protein A, the added antibodies link specifically with the protein A trapped at the bottom of the wells keeping the virus antibodies in a specific orientation so that the F(ab´)2 portion of the antibodies will be free to trap the virus particles. The F(ab´)2 portion of the virus antibody orientation will increase the sensitivity of the PAS- ELISA by increasing the proportion of appropriately aligned antibody molecules. The exposed virus particles will link to the F(ab´)2 portion of a second added layer of the same antibodies which will be detected by an enzyme-conjugated protein A followed by colorimetric changes of a specific substrate that is added into the wells (Figure 5B).

3.1.5 Immune Precipitation ELISA (IP- ELISA)

Considering the problems with plant viruses whose particles are not well adsorbed in the ELISA plate wells, a new ELISA technique involving the immune virus particle precipitation (IP- ELISA) was developed and validated for detection of plant viruses from different families and genera, especially those from the genus *Comovirus* (Lima et al., 2011b). As for the other ELISA procedures, approximately 0.5 g of virus infected plant tissues are ground in ELISA extraction buffer and 0.5 ml from the obtained extract is mixed with an equal volume of specific antiserum diluted to 1:100 to 1:1000 (v/v). The mixture of infected plant extract and the antiserum is incubated at 37 °C for 3 h or overnight at 4 °C and centrifuged at 5,000 g for 10 min. The pellet containing the virus particles linked to the antibodies are ressuspended in ELISA extraction buffer and used as for conventional indirect ELISA (Figure 6). The IP- ELISA showed efficiency for detection of virus from different families and genera in different kinds of infected tissues. The immune virus precipitation followed by ELISA (IP- ELISA) for detection of viruses was shown to be a sensitive and practical diagnostic technique for plant viruses, especially for *Cowpea severe mosaic virus* (CPSMV) and *Squash mosaic virus* (SQMV), family *Comoviridae*, genus *Comovirus* (Lima *et al.*, 2011b), whose virus particles do not adsorb well in the bottom of the plate wells (personal observation). This method increases the efficiency of the indirect ELISA (Figure 7) without the necessity of using protein A.

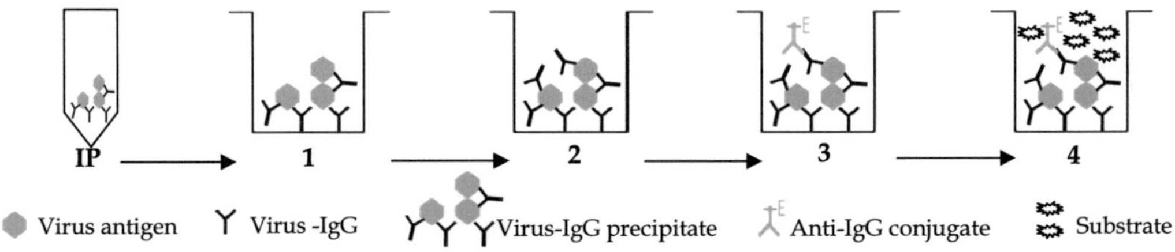

Fig. 6. Diagrammatic drawings of immune precipitation enzyme-linked immunosorbent assay (IP- ELISA) for detection of plant virus with particles that do not adhere well in the ELISA plates.

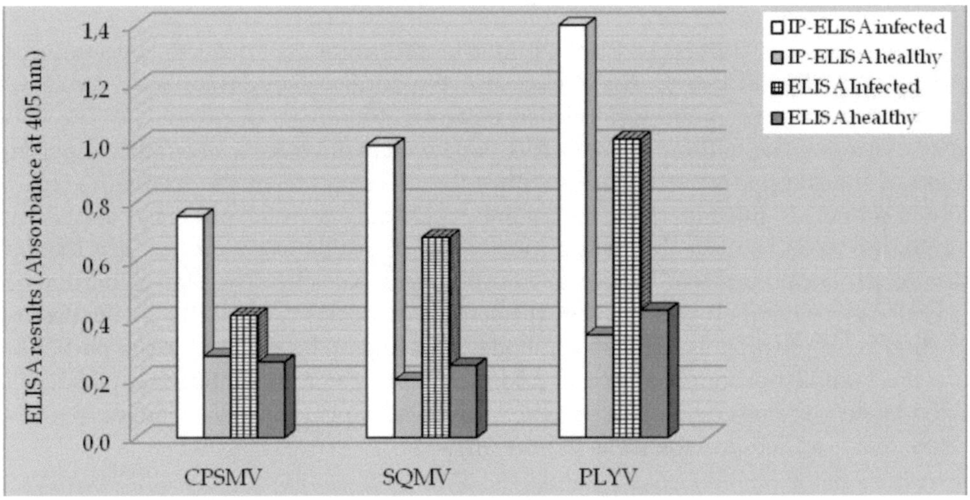

Fig. 7. Results showing the sensitivities of immune precipitation ELISA (IP- ELISA) and indirect ELISA for detection of *Cowpea severe mosaic virus* (CPSMV), *Squash mosaic virus* (SQMV) and *Papaya lethal yellowing virus* (PLYV) in infected tissues.

3.1.6 Rapid immunochromatographic tests for field and laboratory diagnosis

In recent years rapid serological tests using lateral flow immunochromatography have been developed for plant virus diagnosis (Tsuda et al., 1992; Ward et al., 2004). Samples can be analyzed in the field or the laboratory in less than 30 minutes. In one form of the test, strips containing virus-specific antibodies are placed in extracts from plants to be assayed, and the sample wicks upward. If virus is present, it reacts with specific antibody to give a visible band at the test line on the strip, which indicates a positive result. Such tests have shown good agreement with results obtained by conventional ELISA tests (Agdia, 2007a; 2007b). Variations of the immunochromatographic tests for certain plant viruses are available commercially, eg., at Agdia, Bioreba, or Forsite Diagnostics (Pocket Diagnostic).

3.1.7 Immune Capture Polymerase Chain Reaction (IC-PCR)

A technique called immune capture polymerase chain reaction (IC-PCR), which combines the technical advantages of PCR with the practical advantages of serology, was developed for the detection of several different plant viruses (Nolasco et al., 1993). First, microtiter tubes are coated with specific virus antibodies and incubated at 37°C for 2 h. After washing, the microtiter tubes coated with the antibodies will trap the virus particles which will be disrupted followed by the release of viral nucleic acid. The virus nucleic acid is amplified by polymerase chain reaction (PCR) or reverse transcription PCR (RT- PCR), and the entire procedure is carried out in a single microtiter tube (Figure 8A). According to Nolasco et al. (1993) this method also can be used with monoclonal antibodies raised to double-stranded RNA permitting the possibility of detection of satellite-RNAs or viroids. The IC-PCR has been shown to be a very useful alternative in virus detection from plant material and insect vectors (Candresse et al., 1998; Mumford & Seal, 1997; Mulholland, 2009; Wetzel et al., 1992).

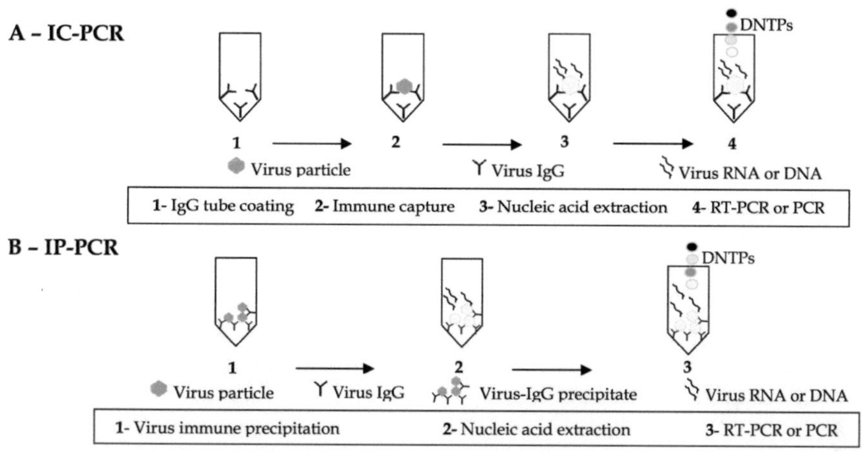

Fig. 8. Diagrammatic drawings of immune capture polymerase chain reaction IC-PCR (A) and immune precipitation polymerase chain reaction IP-PCR (B) for plant virus detection.

3.2 Immune Precipitation Polymerase Chain Reaction (IP-PCR)

A new PCR technology involving virus particles immune precipitation (IP-PCR) was developed for identification and molecular characterization of plant viruses from different families and genera (Lima et al., 2011a). The new technique is very practical, specific and minimizes problems with RNA extraction combining the serological properties and the technical advantages of virus nucleic acid amplification (Figure 8B). Approximately 0.5 g of plant tissues infected with virus are grind in 1.0 ml of extraction buffer (0.15 M Na_2CO_3, 0.035 M of $NaHCO_3$ and 0.007 M of sodium diethyldithiocarbamate, pH 9.6). The extract is obtained by straining through triple cheesecloth, and 0.5 ml was mixed with an equal volume of specific virus polyclonal antiserum diluted to 1:500 (v/v) in the antiserum buffer (PBS-Tween 20 with 0.5 M polyvinylpyrrolidone, 0.2% ovalbumin, 0.03 M sodium azide, 0.17% of sodium diethyldithiocarbamate). The mixture is incubated at 37 °C for 3 h or overnight at 4 °C, and centrifuged at 5,000 g for 10 min. The precipitated virus particles linked with their specific antibodies are disrupted for RNA extraction using Trizol® Reagent according to the manufacturer's instructions. Alternatively the virus RNA is extracted with a RNA isolation system (Promega, Madison, WI). A first strand cDNA is synthesized from each virus RNA using their antisense specific primers and the M-MLV Reverse Transcriptase (Promega, Madison, WI). The cDNA fragments corresponding to virus RNA are amplified by PCR. This newly developed immune virus precipitation followed by PCR or RT-PCR (IP-PCR) was shown to be a practical and sensitive technique for detection of plant viruses. Similar to IC-PCR, the IP-PCR has the advantage of combining the analyses of the serological and the molecular virus properties. Additionally, the IP-PCR technique reduces the risk of cross-contamination with plant RNAs and does not require expensive equipment and reagents. The application of the new IP-PCR technology for detection of virus in infected plant tissues has been useful for all the virus-host combinations tested so far. The new IP-PCR technique provides partial virus particle purification by its specific immune precipitation, and it should be especially useful for detecting viruses that are present in low or variable titers in plant species which contain various forms of PCR amplification inhibitors. The method has the typical sensitivity of assays based on PCR combined with the virus serological properties and is not more laborious than ELISA procedures.

The IP-PCR was shown to be capable of detecting the presence of RNA of Papaya lethal yellowing virus (PLYV) up to dilution of 1:10,000 of the infected plant extracts and did not amplify any cDNA from healthy plant extracts (Figure 9). The new technique also was demonstrated to be efficient for detecting the presence of five virus species from three different families: Bromoviridae, Comoviridae, Potyviridae and Sobemoviridae (Lima et al., 2011a). In addition to its sensitivity and specificity, similar to IC-PCR (Nolasco et al., 1993; Mumford & Seal, 1997; Candresse et al., 1998), the IP-PCR has the advantage of combining the analyses of the serological and the molecular virus properties. Additionally, the IP-PCR technique reduces the risk of cross-contamination with plant RNAs and does not require expensive equipment and reagents.

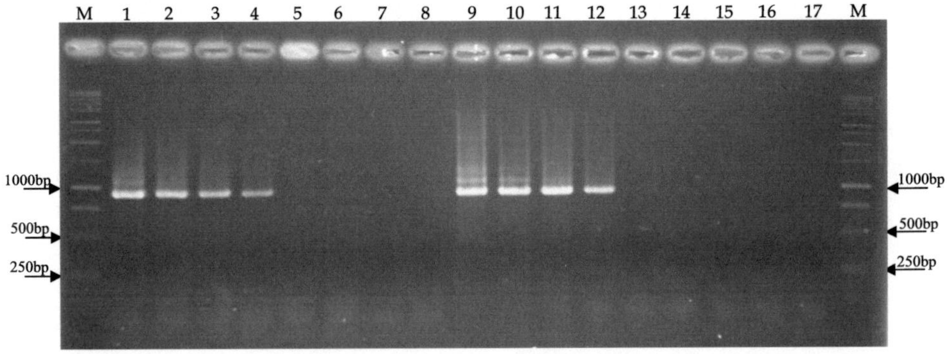

Fig. 9. Results of reverse transcription polymerase chain reaction (RT-PCR) and immune precipitation PCR (IP-PCR) of plant tissues infected with *Papaya lethal yellowing virus* (PLYV) at different dilutions of the plant extracts. Lanes 1-4: RT-PCR of PLYV infected papaya in the dilutions of 1:10 (1), 1:100 (2), 1:1,000 (3) and 1:10,000 (4); Lanes 5-8: RT-PCR of healthy papaya in the correspondent dilutions; Lanes 9-12: IP-RT-PCR of PLYV infected papaya in the dilutions of 1:10 (9), 1:100 (10), 1:1,000 (11) and 1:10,000 (12); Lanes 13-17: IP-RT-PCR of healthy papaya in the correspondent dilutions and Lane M: DNA ladder with standards of indicated length in Kb. The gels were stained with ethidium bromide analyzed under UV light.

3.3 Immunoblotting methods

Serological solid support matrix methods similar to ELISA techniques were developed in which the virus antigens are trapped onto a membrane rather than in a microtitre plate. Similar to indirect ELISA, virus particles or their proteins are immobilized on nitrocellulose or nylon membranes (Almeida, 2001; Purcifull et al., 2001). As distinguished from indirect ELISA, it is not necessary to use an ELISA reader for detecting the virus antibodies interactions and for this reason it is not possible to quantify the results by numerical absorbance values (Almeida, 2001; Astier et al., 2007). According to the process by which the virus antigens are applied in the membranes these methods can be divided into three categories: a) Western blot; b) Dot blot or dot immuno binding assay (DIBA) and c) Tissue blot immuno assay (TIBA).

3.3.1 Western blot

In this method the virus protein antigens are transferred from polyacrylamide gels in which they were previously separated by electrophoresis to nitrocellulose or nylon membranes. Several methods can be used to transfer the virus protein and the electro-blotting is the most used system. Similar to ELISA techniques, the proteins are detected in the membrane by the use of specific enzyme labeled antibodies (Almeida, 2001; Purcifull et al., 2001). Different antibody labeling systems, including biotin-avidin and chemiluminescent systems are sometimes used to increase sensitivity. The Western blot is usually used for characterization of virus proteins rather than for detection since it has the advantage of determining the serological and molecular properties of the virus protein.

3.3.2 Dot Blot or Dot Immuno Binding Assay (DIBA)

Although based on the Western blot principle, the dot immunoblotting assay (DIBA) requires a simple and easier method to prepare and apply the samples on nitrocellulose or nylon membranes (Almeida, 2001; Astier et al., 2007; Purcifull et al., 2001). The samples containing the virus antigens are prepared by grinding tissues in Tris-buffered saline and the extracts are applied directly on the membrane. The sample application on the membrane is usually accomplished through the use of a plastic mold with 96 wells which presses the membrane marking the places where the samples should be applied. Usually the spaces not occupied by the antigens on the membrane are blocked with neutral protein solution. The addition of virus IgG produced in rabbit and the anti-rabbit IgG produced in mouse follow protocols similar to indirect ELISA or PTA-ELISA (Figure 3), except that the positive reactions in DIBA are recorded as colored dots on the membrane. Considering that DIBA is a simple, less laborious and quick test, it can be used routinely for plant virus indexing and survey programs (Almeida, 2001; Astier et al., 2007; Banttari & Goodwin, 1985; Graddon & Randles, 1986; Heide & Lange, 1988; Lange & Heide, 1986; Makkouk et al., 1993; Purcifull et al., 2001; Rybicki & Von Wechmar, 1982). One disadvantage of DIBA is the possibility of sap components interfering with the antigen-antibody reactions, resulting in subsequent problems with the diagnostic results.

3.3.3 Tissue Blot Immune Assay (TIBA)

This is the simplest immunoblotting assay technique developed for virus antigen detection in different types of plant and insect tissues. It is a variation of DIBA in which the samples consist of preparation of infected plant tissues. The tissue immunoblotting assay (TIBA) can be used to detect virus antigens in plant tissues such as leaf, stem, bulb, tuber, root and fruit or insect vectors of plant viruses. The tissues are cut with razor blades and pressed on the membrane to transfer the virus particles or protein (Hsu & Lawson, 1991; Makkouk et al., 1993; Navot et al., 1989; Polston et al., 1991; Purcifull et al., 2001). The detection of the virus antigens applied on the membrane is accomplished by protocols similar to those used for indirect ELISA or PTA-ELISA (Figure 3) and for DIBA. As with DIBA, sometimes the sap components can interfere with the diagnostic results and the color of the sap interferes with the observation of weak virus antigen antibody reactions. The TIBA technique has been demonstrated to be sensitive enough to evaluate the *in situ* distribution of plant virus species from different families and genera (Astier et al., 2007; Makkouk et. al., 1993). As with DIBA the virus-antibody interactions are not quantified since the results are not presented by numerical forms by absorbance values as in the ELISA variations (Almeida, 2001; Astier et al., 2007). The low cost and simplicity of these immunoblotting assay techniques (DIBA and TIBA) make them useful for laboratories with limited facilities (Astier et. al., 2007; Makkouk & Kumari, 2002). Another advantage of these methods is that the samples can be blotted onto the membranes right in the field or in simple laboratories and shipped for further processing at a more equipped laboratory (Naidu & Hughes, 2001).

3.4 Serologically specific electron microscopy

A technique known as serologically specific electron microscopy (SSEM) was introduced by Derrick (1973) and it has become widely used in plant virology (Derrick & Brlansky, 1976; Lima & Purcifull, 1980; Milne, 1991; Naidu & Hughes, 2001). This technique combines the specificity of serological properties with the morphology of the virus particles visualized in the electron microscope. Virus particles are selectively trapped on antibody-coated grids with little contaminating host-plant material (Lima & Purcifull., 1980). Copper electron microscope grids coated preferably with parlodion film are treated with the virus specific antiserum diluted to 1:1,000 - 1:6,000 in an appropriate buffer. The antibody coated grids are washed with buffer and floated on drops of extracts from virus infected plant tissue at room temperature for 3 - 4 h. After washing again for three times, the grids are stained with 1.0% uranyl acetate in 50% ethanol, dried and examined in the electron microscope (Figure 10).

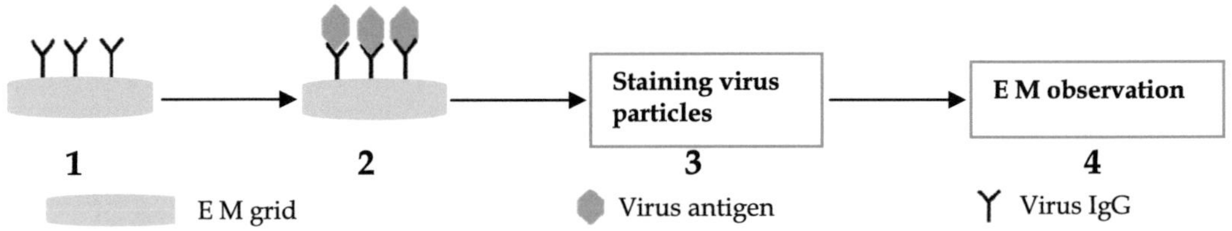

Fig. 10. Diagrammatic drawings of serologically specific electron microscopy (SSEM) for detection of plant virus.

This technique has been used to detect polyhedral and rod shaped virus (Figure 11). It has the great advantage of requiring only very small amounts of antiserum and antigens, and does not require the use of labeled antibodies. For those reason, the SSEM technique is more sensitive for detecting virus particles in leaf extracts than the leaf dip method and shows little contaminating host-plant material (Figure 11; Lima & Purcifull., 1980). Other advantages are that polyclonal antiserum can be used without interfering in the virus particle observations and samples can be blotted onto the IgG coated grids in one small laboratory and shipped for further analysis in an electron microscope Center. Considering the requirement of an electron microscope, the SSEM is recommended for confirmatory tests using small numbers of samples. Some variations of the SSEM have been developed including the decoration of virus particles (Purcifull et al., 2001).

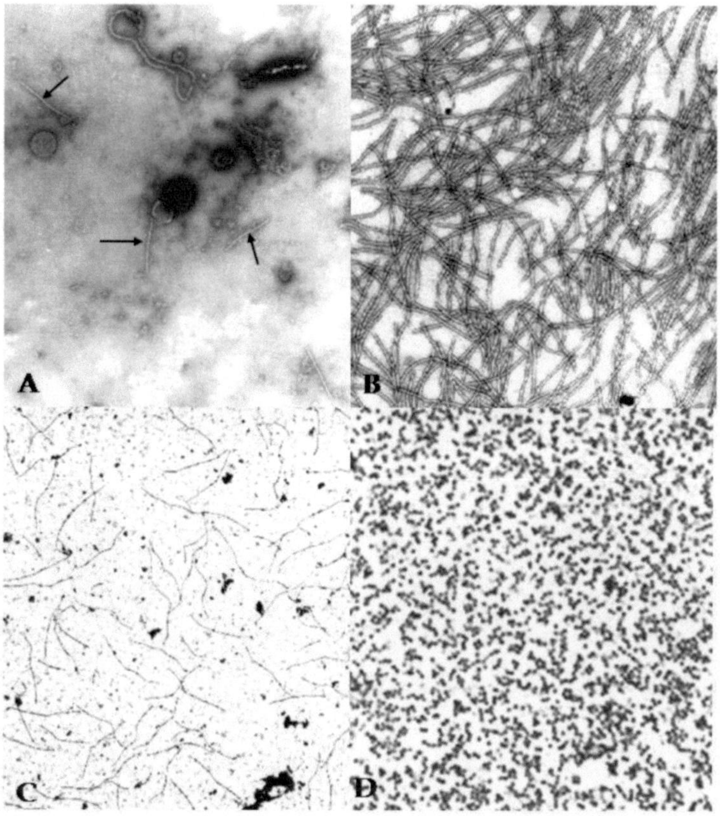

Fig. 11. Electron micrographs of virus particles in the transmission electron microscope. A) Leaf dip preparation with *Blackeye cowpea mosaic virus* (BlCMV) negatively stained with phosphotungstic acid (arrows indicate virus particles); B) Purified BlCMV particles negatively stained with phosphotungstic acid; C) BlCMV particles on grids sensitized with antibodies for BlCMV according to the method for serologically specific electron microscopy (SSEM), and positively stained with uranyl acetate and D) Hexagonal particles of *Cowpea mosaic virus* (CPMV) on grids sensitized with antibodies for CPMV according to the SSEM technique, positively stained with uranyl acetate.

3.5 Double immunodiffusion

The double immunodiffusion test in agar gel also known as the Ouchterlony test (Ouchterlony, 1962) is based in the fact that the antigens and the antibodies deposited into wells opened in agar gels diffuse in all directions through the medium. This test is preferentially developed in Petri dishes but it can also be accomplished on microscope slides. Reactant wells are opened in the agar gel with cork borers or adjustable gel cutting device and the agar plugs are removed with glass tubing connected to a vacuum pump. A useful gel pattern consists of up to six peripheral antigen wells of 3 to 7 mm in diameter, surrounding a central serum well. Each peripheral well is 4 to 5 mm from the central well at the closest point (Figure 12). The antigens are pipetted into the peripheral wells and the antiserum into the central well. Reactions usually appear within 12 h and are complete within 24 -48 h after the addition of the reactants. The results can be viewed and recorded photographically by dark-field illumination (Purcifull & Batchelor, 1977).

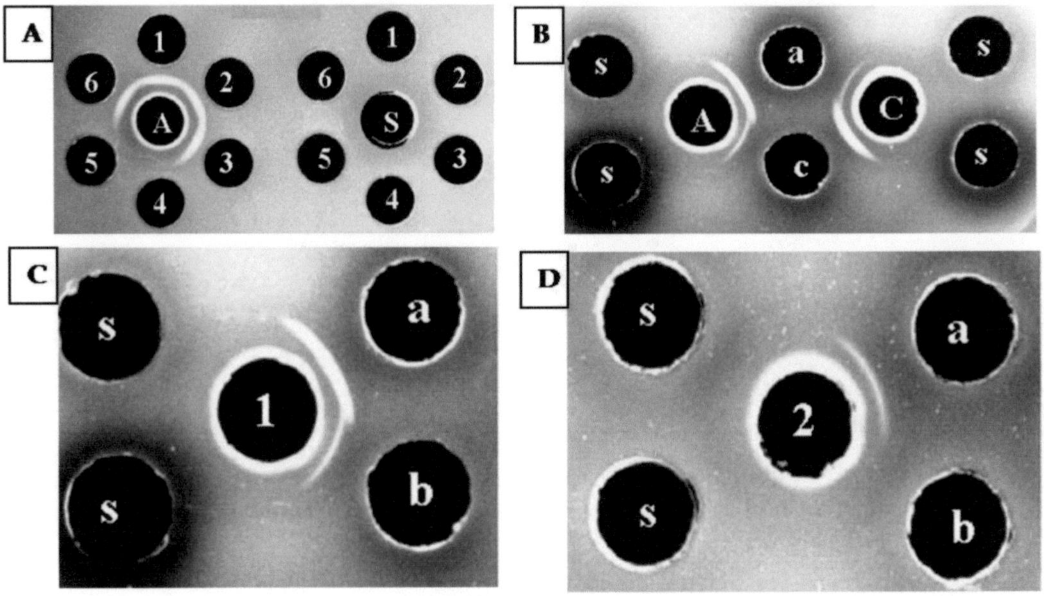

Fig. 12. Serological double immune diffusion test in agar gel: A) A hexagonal arrangement with the antigens in peripheral wells and the antiserum (A) and normal serum (S) in the central well; extracts of infected plants (1, 2, 3 and 6) and extracts from healthy plant (4 and 5); B) Reciprocal tests with antisera to: (A) *Blackeye cowpea mosaic virus* (BlCMV) and (C) *Bean common mosaic virus* (BCMV) , showing spur formation between the virus antigens; C, D) Intra-gel cross absorption tests with BlCMV (C) and with BCMV (D): (1) antiserum for BlCMV, (2) extracts of plants infected with BCMV and 12 h later antiserum for BlCMV; (a) extracts of plants infected with BlCMV, (b) extracts of plants infected with BCMV and (s) extracts of healthy plants.

Depending on the medium composition this method can be used for polyhedral or rod shaped viruses. Although the polyhedral particles of 28 to 40 nm could diffuse through the medium pores, the long rod shaped viruses over 300 nm need to be dissociated into their coat protein units to diffuse through the medium (Purcifull & Batchelor, 1977; Purcifull et al., 2001; Almeida & Lima, 2001). This can be accomplished by the use of several chemical compounds, especially sodium dodecyl sulfate (SDS). Although not very sensitive this test is still preferred to evaluate the antiserum titers, for routine diagnosis of a few samples and to study the serological relationship among some plant viruses. Using reciprocal double immunodiffusion tests with polyclonal antisera, Oliveira et al. (2000) confirmed the type of serological relationship among PRSV-W, WMV and ZYMV demonstrated by indirect ELISA.

The intra-gel cross absorption test is a variation of the standard double immunodiffusion technique recommended to define the serological relationship among virus species or strains. It is still used to define the relationship among virus species and isolates from the genera *Potyvirus* and *Comovirus*. To develop this method, very highly concentrated extracts of heterologous viruses are deposited into the central well 12 h before the antiserum and the homologous virus are pipetted into their respective wells (Figure 12).

5. Acknowledgments

We thank the Foundation for Scientific and Technological Development of the State of Ceará (FUNCAP) and the National Council for Scientific and Technological Development (CNPq) of Brazil for their funding to conduct this research and for the author fellowships.

6. References

Agdia, Inc. (2007a). Agdia announces easy-to-use, on site immunostrip for rapid detection of all strains of Potato virus Y (PVY). In: *Plant Health Progress*, 19 February 2007. ISSN 1535-1025

Agdia, Inc. (2007b). Agdia's easy-to-use, on-site immunostrip identifies hard-to-detect Cymbidium mosaic and Odontoglossum ringspot viruses in orchids. In: *Plant Health Progress*, 4 May 2007. ISSN 1535-1025

Almeida, A.M.R. & Lima, J.A.A. (2001). Técnicas sorológicas aplicadas à fitovirologia, In: *Princípios e técnicas aplicados em fitovirologia*, A.M.R. Almeida & J.A.A. Lima, (Eds.), 33-62, Edições Sociedade Brasileira Fitopatologia, ISBN 901648, Fortaleza, Ceará, Brazil

Almeida, A.M.R. (2001). Detecção e quantificação de vírus pelo teste de ELISA, In: *Princípios e técnicas aplicados em fitovirologia*, edited by A.M.R. Almeida & J.A.A. Lima, (Eds.), 63-94, Edições Sociedade Brasileira Fitopatologia, ISBN 901648, Fortaleza, Ceará, Brazil

Astier, S.; Albouy, J.; Maury, Y.; Robaglia, C. & Lecoq, H. (2007). *Principles of Plant Virology: Genome, pathogenicity, virus ecology*, Science Publishers, ISBN: 1578083168, New Hampshire, USA

Baker, C. A.; Lecoq, H. & Purcifull, D. E. (1991). Serological and biological variability among papaya ringspot virus type-W isolates in Florida. *Phytopathology*, Vol. 81, No. 7, (July 1991), pp.722-728, ISSN 0031-949X

Banttari, E.E. & Goodwin, P.H. (1985). Detection of potato viruses S, X, and Y by enzyme-linked immunosorbent assay on nitrocellulose membranes (dot-ELISA). *Plant Disease*, Vol.69, No.3, (March 1985), pp.202–205, ISSN: 0191-2917

Barbosa, F. R. & Paguio, D. R. (1982). Vírus da Mancha Anelar do Mamoeiro: Incidência e Efeito na produção do mamoeiro, *Fitopatologia Brasileira*, Vol.7, No.3, (July 1982), pp.365-373, ISSN 01004158

Bezerra, D.R.; Lima, J.A.A. & Xavier-Filho, J. (1995). Purificação e caracterização de um isolado cearense do vírus do endurecimento dos frutos do maracujazeiro, *Fitopatologia Brasileira,* Vol.20, No.4, (December 1995), pp.553-560, ISSN 01004158

Cancino, M.; Abouzid, A. M.; Morales, F. J.; Purcifull, D. E.; Polston, J. E. & Hiebert, E. (1995). Generation and characterization of three monoclonal antibodies useful in detecting and distinguishing bean golden mosaic virus isolates, *Phytopathology,* Vol.85, No.4, (April 1995), pp.484-490, ISSN 0031-949X

Candresse, T.; Hammond, R.W. & Hadidi, A. (1998). Detection and identification of plant viruses and viroids using polymerase chain reaction (PCR), In: *Control of plant virus diseases,* A. Hadidi, R.K. Khetarpal & K. Koganezawa, (Eds.), 399–416, APS Press, ISBN 978-0-89054-191-3, St. Paul, MN, USA

Clark, M.F. & Adams, A.N. (1977). Characteristics of the microplate method of enzyme-linked immunosorbent assay for the detection of plant viruses, *Journal of General Virology,* Vol.34, No.3, (December 1977), pp.475-483, ISSN 00221317

Clark, M.F. & Bar-Joseph, M. (1984). Enzyme immunosorbent assays in plant virology, In *Methods in virology,* K. Maramorosch & H. Koprowski (Eds.), 51–85, Academic Press, ISBN 0124702082, New York, USA

Cooper, J.I. & Edwards, M.L. (1986). Variations and limitations of enzyme-amplified immunoassays, In: *Developments and applications in virus testing,* R.A.C. Jones & L. Torrance, (Eds.), 139–154, Association of Applied Biologists, ISBN 02690713. Wellesbourne, UK

Derrick, K.S. & Brlansky, R.H. (1976). Assay for virus and mycoplasma using serological specific electron microscopy, *Phytopathology,* Vol.66, No.6, (June 1976), pp.815-820, ISSN 0031-949X

Derrick, K.S. (1973). Quantitative assay for plant viruses using serological specific electron microscopy, *Virology,* Vol.56, No.2, (December 1973), pp.652-653, ISSN 0426822

Desbiez, C.; Costa, C.; Wipf-Scheibel, C.; Girard, M. & Lecoq, H. (2007). Serological and molecular variability of watermelon mosaic virus (genus Potyvirus), *Archives of Virology,* Vol.152, No.4, (April 2007), pp.775-781, ISSN: 0304-8608

Florindo, M.I. & Lima, J.A.A. (1991). Danos ocasionados por um potyvirus em *Clitoria ternatea* L. e sua transmissibilidade por ferramentas de corte, *Ciência Agronômica,* Vol.22, No.1/2, (June/December 1991), pp.97-102, ISSN 0045-6888

Graddon, D.J. & Randles, J.W. (1986). Single antibody dot immunoassay: a simple technique for rapid detection of a plant virus, *Journal of Virological Methods,* Vol.13, No.1, (April 1986), pp.63–69, ISSN 0166 0934

Hampton, R.; Ball, E. & De Boer, S. (1990). *Serological methods for detection and identification of viral and bacterial plant pathogens,* American Phytopathological Society, ISBN: 0890541159, St. Paul, MN, USA

Heide, M. & Lange, L. (1988). Detection of potato leafroll virus and potato viruses M,S,X, and Y by dot immunobinding on plain paper, *Potato Research,* Vol.31, No.2, (June 1988), pp.367–373, ISSN 18714528

Hiebert, E.; Purcifull, D. E. & Christie, R. G. (1984). Purification and immunological analyses of plant viral inclusion bodies, In: *Methods in Virology,* Vol. VII. K. Maramorsch & H. Koprowski, (Eds.), 225-280, Academic Press, London, ISBN 0-12-470270-4

Hsu, H.T. & Lawson, R.H. (1991). Direct tissue blotting for detection of tomato spotted wilt virus in *Impatiens, Plant Disease,* Vol.75, No.4, (April 1991), pp.292–295, ISSN: 0191-2917

Lange, L. & Heide, M. (1986). Dot immuno binding (DIB) for detection of virus in seed, *Canadian Journal of Plant Pathology,* Vol.8, No.4, (October 1986), pp.373–379, ISSN 0706-0661

Lima, J. A. A., & Gomes, M. N. S. (1975). Identificação de "papaya ringspot virus" no Ceará, *Fitossanidade,* Vol.1, No.2, (June 1975), pp.56-59, ISSN: 01004204

Lima, J.A.A. & Amaral, M.R.G. (1985). Purificação e sorologia de "squash mosaic virus" isolado de melancia, *Fitopatologia Brasileira,* Vol.10, No.3, (June 1985), pp.605-611, ISSN 01004158

Lima, J.A.A. & Nelson, M.R. (1977). Etiology and epidemiology of mosaic of cowpea in Ceará, Brasil, *Plant Disease Reporter,* Vol.61, No.10 , (October 1977), pp.864-867, ISSN 00320811

Lima, J.A.A. & Purcifull, D.E. (1980). Immunochemical and microscopical techniques for detecting blackeye cowpea mosaic and soybean mosaic viruses in hypocotyls of germinated seeds, *Phytopathology,* Vol.70, No.2, (February 1980), pp.142-147, ISSN: 0031-949X

Lima, J.A.A., Purcifull, D.E. & Hiebert, E. (1979). Purification, partial characterization, and serology of blackeye cowpea mosaic virus, *Phytopathology,* Vol.69, No.12, (December 1979), pp.1252-1258, ISSN: 0031-949X

Lima, J.A.A.; Florindo, M.I. & Kitajima, E.W. (1993). Some properties of a potyvirus isolated from *Clitoria ternatea, Fitopatologia Brasileira,* Vol.18, No.2, (June 1993), pp.213-218, ISSN 01004158

Lima, J.A.A.; Lima, A.R.T. & Marques, M.A.L. (1994). Purificação e caracterização sorológica de um isolado do vírus do amarelo letal do mamoeiro 'solo' obtido no Ceará, *Fitopatologia Brasileira,* Vol.19, No.3, (September 1994), pp.437-441, ISSN 01004158

Lima, J.A.A.; Nascimento, A.K.Q.; Radaelli, P.; Silva, A.K.F. & Silva, F.R. (2011a). Immune precipitation polymerase chain reaction for identification of plant viruses, *Proceedings of XXII Proceedings of XXII National Meeting of Virology,* Vol. 16, Suplement 1, p. 56, (October 2011), ISSN 5192563, Atibaia, SP

Lima, J.A.A.; Nascimento, A.K.Q.; Silva, F.R.; Silva, A.K.F. & Aragão, M.L. (2011b). An immune precipitation enzyme-linked immunosorbent (IP-ELISA) technique for identification of plant viruses, *Proceedings of XXII National Meeting of Virology,* Vol. 16, Suplement 1, p. 56, (October 2011), ISSN 5192563, Atibaia, SP

Lima, J.A.A.; Silveira, L.F.S.; Santos, C.D.G. & Gonçalves, M.F.B. (1991). Infecção natural em gergelim ocasionada por um potyvirus, *Fitopatologia Brasileira,* Vol.16, No.1, (March 1991), pp.60-62, ISSN 01004158

Lima, J.A.A.; Sittolin, I.M. & Lima, R.C.A. (2005). Diagnose e estratégias de controle de doenças ocasionadas por vírus, In: *Feijão caupi: Avanços tecnológicos,* F.R. Freire Filho, J.A.A. Lima; Silva P.H.S & V.Q Ribeiro, (Eds.), 404-459, Embrapa Informação Tecnológica, ISSN: 85-7383-283-5, Brasília, Brazil

Lima, R. C. A.; Lima, J. A. A.; Souza Jr., M. T.; Pio-Ribeiro, G. & Andrade, G. P. (2001). Etiologia e estratégias de controle de viroses do mamoeiro no Brasil, *Fitopatologia Brasileira,* Vol.26, No.4, (December 2001), pp.689-702, ISSN 01004158

Makkouk, K.M. & Kumari, S.G. (2002). Low-cost paper can be used in tissue-blot immunoassay for detection of cereal and legume viruses, *Phytopathologia Mediterranea*, Vol.41, No.3, (December 2002), pp.275-278, ISSN 0031-9465

Makkouk, K.M.; Hsu, H.T. & Kumari, S.G. (1993). Detection of three plant viruses by dot-blot and tissue-blot immunoassays using chemiluminescent and chromogenic substrates, *Journal of Phytopathology*, Vol.139, No.2, (October 1993), pp.97–102, ISSN 09311785

Marciel-Zambolim, E.; Kunieda-Alonso, S.; Matsuoka, K.; Carvalho, M. G. & Zerbini, F. M. (2003). Purification and some properties of Papaya meleira virus, a novel virus infecting papayas in Brazil, *Plant Pathology*, Vol.52, No.3, (March 2003), pp.389-394, ISSN 13653059

Milne, R.G. (1991). Immunoelectron microscopy for virus identification, In: *Electron microscopy of plant pathogens*, K. Mendgen & D.E. Lesemann, (Eds.), 87–120, Springer-Verlag, ISBN 038752777X, Berlin, Germany

Moura, M.C.C.L.; Lima, J.A.A.; Oliveira, V.B. & Gonçalves, M.F.B. (2001). Identificação sorológica de espécies de vírus que infetam cucurbitáceas em áreas produtoras do Maranhão, *Fitopatologia Brasileira*, Vol.26, No.1, (March 2001), pp.90-92, ISSN 01004158

Mulholland, V. (2009). Immunocapture-PCR for Plant Virus Detection, In: *Plant Pathology: Techniques and Protocols*, Robert Burns, (Ed.), 183-192, Scottish Agricultural Science Agency, ISBN: 1588297993, Edinburgh EH12 9FJ, UK

Mumford, R.A. & Seal, S.E. (1997). Rapid single-tube immunocapture RT-PCR for the detection of two yam potyviruses, *Journal of Virological Methods*, Vol.69, No.1/2, (December 1997), pp.73–79, ISSN: 0166-0934

Naidu, R.A. & Hughes, J.d'A. (2001). Methods for the detection of plant virus diseases, In: *Plant virology in sub-Saharan Africa*, J.d'A. Hughes & B. O. Odu, (Eds.), 233–260, Proceedings of a Conference Organized by IITA, International Institute of Tropical Agriculture, ISBN 9781312149, Nigeria

Nascimento, A. K. Q.; Lima, J.A.A.; Nascimento, A.L.L.; Beserra Jr., J.A.B. & Purcifull, D. E. (2010). Biological, physical, and molecular properties of a *Papaya lethal yellowing virus* isolate, *Plant Disease*, Vol.94, No.10, (October 2010), pp.1206-1212, ISSN: 0191-2917

Nascimento, A. K. Q.; Radaelli, P.; Lima, J.A.A. & Silva, F.R. (2011). Indirect enzyme linked immunosorbent assay and polymerase chain reaction for detection of viruses in banana tissues, In: *Proceedings of 44º Congresso Brsileiro de Fitopatologia*, Vol. 36, p.612, (August 2011), ISBN 19825676, Bento Gonçalves, RS

Navot, N., Ber, R. & Czosnek, H. (1989). Rapid detection of tomato yellow leaf curl virus in squashes of plants and insect vectors, *Phytopathology*, Vol.79, No.5, (May 1989), pp.562–568, ISSN: 0031-949X

Nolasco, G.; Blas, C. de; Torres, V. & Ponz, F. (1993). A method combining immunocapture and PCR amplification in a microtiter plate for the detection of plant viruses and subviral pathogens, *Journal of Virological Methods*, Vol.45, No.2, (December 1993), pp.201–218, ISSN: 0166-0934

Oliveira, V.B.; Lima, J.A.A.; Vale, C.C. & Paiva, W.O. (2000). Caracterização biológica e sorológica de isolados de potyvirus obtidos de cucurbitáceas no Nordeste brasileiro, *Fitopatologia Brasileira,* Vol.25, No.4, (October 2000), pp.628-636, ISSN 01004158

Oliveira, V.B.; Queiroz, M.A. & Lima, J.A.A. (2002). Fontes de resistência aos principais potyvirus isolados de cucurbitáceas no Nordeste brasileiro, *Horticultura Brasileira,* Vol.20, No.4, (December 2000), pp.589-592, ISSN 0102-0536

Ouchterlony, O. (1962). Diffusion-in-gel methods for immunological analysis II, *Progress in Allergy,* Vol.6, No.5, (September 1962), pp.30–154, ISSN: 0079-6034

Polston, J.E.; Burbrick, P. & Perring, T.M. (1991). Detection of plant virus coat proteins on whole leaf blots, *Analytical Biochemistry,* Vol.196, No.2, (August 1991), pp.267–270, ISSN: 0003-2697

Purcifull, D. E.; Hiebert, E.; Petersen, M. & Webb, S. (2001). Virus detection - Serology, In: *Encyclopedia of Plant Pathology,* O. C. Maloy & T. D. Murray, (Eds.), Vol. 2, 1100-1109, John Wiley & Sons, Inc. ISBN: 0-471-29817-4

Purcifull, D.E. & Batchelor, D.L. (1977). *Immunodiffusion tests with sodium dodecyl sulfate (SDS) - treated plant viruses and plant virus inclusions.* University of Florida Agric. Exp. Stn. Bull. N° 788, ASIN B0006WMAKA, Florida, USA

Rabelo Filho, F.A.C.; Lima, J.A.A.; Ramos, N.F.; Gonçalves, M.F.B. & Carvalho, K.F. (2005). Produção de anti-soro para o vírus do mosaico da abóbora mediante imunização oral de coelhos, *Revista Ciência Agronômica,* Vol. 36, No.3, (October/December 2005), pp.344-347, ISSN 0045-6888

Rybicki, E.P. & Von Wechmar, M.B.. (1982). Enzyme-assisted immune detection of plant virus proteins electroblotted onto nitrocellulose paper, *Journal of Virological Methods,* Vol.5, No.5-6, (December 1982), pp.267–278, ISSN: 0166-0934

Torrance, L. (1992). Serological methods to detect plant viruses: production and use of monoclonal antibodies, In: *Techniques for the rapid detection of plant pathogens,* J.M. Duncan & L. Torrance, (Eds.), 7–33, Blackwell Scientific Publications, ISBN: 0632030666, Oxford, UK.

Tsuda, S.; Kameya-Iwaki, M.; Hanada, K.; Kouda, Y.; Hikata, M. & Tomaru, K. (1992). A novel detection and identification technique for plant viruses: rapid immunofilter paper assay (RIPA), *Plant Disease,* Vol.76, No.5, (May 1992), pp.466-469, ISSN: 0191-2917

Van Regenmortel, M.H.V. & Dubs, M.C. (1993). Serological procedures, In: *Diagnosis of plant virus diseases,* R.E.F. Matthews (Ed.), 159–214, CRC Press, Boca Raton, ISBN:0849342848, Florida, USA.

Van Regenmortel, M.H.V. (1982). *Serology and immunochemistry of plant viruses,* Academic Press, ISBN-10: 0127141804, New York, USA

Ventura, J. A.; Costa, H. & Tatagiba, J. S. (2004). Papaya diseases and integrated control Pages. In: *Diseases of fruits and vegetables: diagnosis and management,* Naqvi, (Ed.), 201-268, Dordrecht: Kluwer Academic Publishers, ISBN: 1402018231

Voller, A.A.; Bartlett, A.; Bidwell, D.E.; Clark, M.F. & Adams, A.N. (1976). The detection of viruses by enzyme-linked immunosorbent assay (ELISA), *Journal of General Virology,* Vol.33, No. 1, (October 1976), pp.165-167, ISSN: 0022-1317

Ward, E.; Foster, S. J.; Fraaije, B. A. & McCartney, H. A. (2004). Plant pathogen diagnostics: immunological and nucleic acid-based approaches, *Annals of Applied Biology,* Vol.145, No.1, (August 2004), pp.1-16, ISSN: 17447348

Wetzel, T.; Candresse, T.; Macquaire, G.; Ravelonandro M.& Dunez, J. (1992). A highly sensitive immunocapture polymerase chain reaction method for plum pox potyvirus detection, *Journal of Virological Methods,* Vol.39, No.1-2 , (September 1992), pp.27–37, ISSN: 0166-0934

Part 3

Serological Diagnosis of Parasitological Diseases

7

Immunodiagnosis of Human Toxocariasis

William H. Roldán[1] and Guita Rubinsky-Elefant[2]
[1]Instituto de Medicina Tropical 'Daniel A. Carrión', Universidad Nacional Mayor de San Marcos, Lima-Perú,
[2]Instituto de Medicina Tropical de São Paulo, Universidade de São Paulo, SP, Brasil

1. Introduction

Human toxocariasis is a helminthic zoonosis caused by larval stages of *Toxocara canis* and, less frequently, by *T. cati*, the roundworms of dogs and cats, respectively. Accidentally, humans ingest embryonated eggs containing the infective larva which are released in the upper small intestine and then pass through the intestinal epithelium to reach the blood vessels, where they can migrate to the different visceral organs and tissues of the body (Despommier, 2003).

An interesting phenomenon is that these parasites cannot develop into adult forms in humans and are restricted to larval forms, migrating through the soft tissues for months and even years and causing local or systemic inflammatory reactions in the affected organ. Sometimes the immune system can even kill the parasite, however, the immunity generated with the first infection fails to protect against future reinfections. It has been reported that the larvae can survive for many years and even decades in the human host, causing local tissue necrosis, eosinophilic inflammatory reactions and granuloma formation (Schantz & Glickman, 1978; ; Minvielle et al., 1999; Magnaval et al., 2001; Despommier, 2003).

The spectrum of the clinical manifestations in human toxocariasis varies widely from asymptomatic cases to systemic infections. Clinical manifestations and the course of the disease will be determined by the inoculum, the frequency of reinfection episodes in the patient, the location of migrating larvae in the affected organ, and the host response (Pawlowski, 2001).

However, both the inoculum and the frequency of reinfection episodes cannot be measured directly in humans, but they can be assumed through the frequency of contaminated environments with *Toxocara* spp. eggs or by the proportion of children with habits of geophagy in the area or region studied (Magnaval et al., 2001; Pawlowski, 2001; Smith et al., 2009). Migrating larvae may be identified by means of clinical examination and the use of diagnostic imaging tests in order to looking for granulomas, either in the eye, brain or liver (Despommier, 2003). Even when it cannot be directly observed, the imaging diagnostics proves to be of aid to suspect the causative agent; however, all clinical suspicion should be confirmed by additional laboratorial tests (Chieffi et al., 2009; Rubinsky-Elefant et al., 2010), as discussed below.

2. *Toxocara* and toxocariasis in humans

Toxocariasis is more probable in tropical and subtropical areas and it is considered of higher risk in populations from both periurban and rural areas with poor sanitation, and where the people do not usually deworm their pets (Glickman & Schantz, 1981). However, this concept has been reversed as there are confirmed cases of toxocariasis in people who have never had dogs at home, which has led to an awareness of the environmental contamination with parasitized dog feces, especially in public parks, children playgrounds and streets (Holland et al., 1991; Uga et al., 1996; Habluetzel et al., 2003; Avcioglu & Balkaya, 2011).

Adult stages of *Toxocara canis* and *T. cati* have their habitat in the small intestine of their definitive hosts: the canines and felines. The adult gravid female of the parasites release their eggs in the intestinal lumen, which are then released outside with the feces. *Toxocara* eggs are not immediately infective. The larval development inside the egg varies according to both the humidity and temperature from the environment. With a temperature of 15 - 35°C and a relative humidity of 85%, most of the eggs become infective after 2 to 5 weeks (Glickman et al., 1979; Despommier, 2003). However, with temperatures above 35 °C the egg become inactivated, but if the temperature is below 15 °C, the larval development is slow, but not destroyed (O'Lorcain, 1995). Most of the reviewed literature considers that a *Toxocara* egg become infective when it contain the second larval stage. Nevertheless, some authors have reported that two changes occur inside the egg and, therefore, the infective phase would be the third larval stage (Araujo, 1972; Minvielle et al., 1999).

Dogs and cats become infected with *Toxocara* by either ingesting infective eggs, ingesting tissues from paratenic hosts containing larvae, by transplacental migration of larvae to the developing puppies, by transmamary passage of larvae through the milk in young puppies, or by ingesting immature adults stages present in the vomit or feces of infected puppies (Minvielle et al., 1999; Despommier, 2003).

When infective *Toxocara* eggs are ingested by puppies, the larvae are released in the small intestine and invade the intestinal mucosa, enter the lymphatic or blood vessels and reach the liver within 24 to 48 hours. Through the bloodstream, the larvae reach the heart and lungs, arrive to the alveolar capillaries and then ascend the respiratory tree to reach the pharynx, where they are swallowed. During the migration, the larvae undergo two changes of their body and finally complete the development process to the adult stage in the small intestine. Egg production occurs between 4 and 6 weeks postinfection (Despommier, 2003).

Interestingly, this process do not occurs in dogs older than 6 months because the migrant larvae do not follow the tracheal route and penetrate into the pulmonary veins and are distributed in almost all the body by means of the systemic circulation, especially in the lungs, liver, kidney, skeletal muscles, but also in the brain. This distribution is known as somatic migration where the parasite is restricted to the larval stage and remains dormant for years (Glickman & Schantz, 1983; Overgaauw, 1997).

Toxocara eggs can also be infective for a number of other species different from canines or felines, a phenomenon known as 'paratenesis' (passage of the infective parasite by one or various hosts with no effect on the completion of its life cycle). Paratenic hosts for toxocariasis include earthworms, mice, rats, rabbits, chickens, pigs, pigeons, sheep, and humans. As the larvae remain alive in the paratenic host for years, a predator may become infected when ingest this parasitized tissues. If a predator is a canine or feline, the larvae complete their development in the alimentary tract, but it depends of the age (Minvielle et al., 1999; Magnaval et al., 2001; Despommier, 2003).

Parasitized puppies are the main reservoir of *Toxocara*. The contamination level produced by a female dog and her parasitized puppies in the immediate area of their habitat is very high. If we consider that adult stages of *Toxocara* have an average life of 4 months and each female worm produce about 200,000 eggs per day, and the intestinal worm charge may range from one to hundreds of them, therefore, infected puppies may contaminate the environment with millions of eggs each day (Minvielle et al., 1999; Despommier, 2003).

Humans become infected by accidental ingestion of embryonated *Toxocara* eggs containing the infective third larval stage. The larvae are released in the proximal small intestine, penetrate the mucosa and, through the blood vessels, they reach the portal vein and then, they may migrates through the systemic circulation. The larvae are distributed throughout the body causing hemorrhages, inflammatory process and granulomas. Many larvae seem to remain 'dormant' for many years and then continue their migration. Eventually some of them may be destroyed by the host immune response, while others seem to be protected by encapsulating them (Magnaval et al., 2001; Despommier, 2003).

A large proportion of *Toxocara* infections are either asymptomatic or have nonspecific symptoms. The most frequently involved organs are liver, lungs, brain, eyes, heart, and skeletal muscles. Clinically, the chronic forms of human toxocariasis may be widespread or localized; being the latter the most common and it can also lead to blindness (Pawlowski, 2001; Despommier, 2003).

The clinical manifestations may be divided into an acute phase (usually uncertain and unspecified) and a chronic phase. The acute phase of infection takes place immediately after the larvae penetrate the intestinal epithelium and reach the blood vessels and through them, migrate to the liver, which is the first organ to be affected. The inflammatory response degree of the live will depend on the number of migrating larvae to be ingested by the host, because a small number of larvae can be achieved unnoticed into the portal vein without producing signs. From there, the larvae can travel to other organs like heart, lungs, and kidney, starting the chronic phase of the infection. This migration may also include immunologically privileged organs such as the eye and brain (Pawlowski, 2001; Smith et al., 2009). Larval migration may generates nonspecific symptoms such as myalgia, fever, malaise, and may cause wheezing and airway hyperresponsiveness, especially in children or predisposed people.

The spectrum of clinical manifestations in human toxocariasis varies widely from asymptomatic cases to systemic forms of the disease; probably due to the size of inoculum and the host response against the migrating larvae (Taylor et al., 1988, Pawlovski, 2001). During the larval migration, the larva releases a high content of metabolic antigens that leads to the activation of the host immune system which generates an immunopathogenic mechanism that causes the clinical manifestations of the disease. The immune response against the parasite is mediated in different proportions of either T-helper 1 (Th1) cells (which leads to a granuloma formation) and T-helper 2 (Th2) cells (an increased production of IgE antibodies and eosinophils) (Sugane & Oshima, 1984; Kayes, 1997; Pawlovski, 2001). In this point, allergic, atopic or eosinophil-related manifestations may occur and depend on the type of response of each *Toxocara* infected host.

3. Clinical manifestations of human toxocariasis

Several clinical forms of human toxocariasis have been described, but until moment, few attempts were made to classify the clinical expressions derived from *Toxocara* infections. A proposed classification made by Pawlovski (2001) correlate the observed clinical status, the involvement of immunopathologic mechanisms, the intensity of the serological response, and the location of *Toxocara* larvae. This new classification divides human toxocariasis into four major forms namely: systemic, compartmentalized, covert and asymptomatic. However, Smith et al. (2009) still consider that human toxocariasis should be classified in three major forms: visceral larva migrans, ocular toxocariasis, and covert toxocariasis.

Visceral larva migrans, described by Beaver et al. (1952), is a severe systemic form of toxocariasis which is characterized by high eosinophilia, hepatosplenomegaly, pulmonary involvement, fever, hypergammaglobulinaemia, and elevated isohemagglutinins. Cases of LMV are uncommon and occur almost exclusively in children (Schantz & Glickman, 1978; Magnaval et al., 2001; Despommier, 2003). However, this syndrome may be restricted to clinically much less severe cases, in which only some signs of the classic visceral larva migrans form may occur, such as hepatomegaly and eosinophilia (Pawlovski, 2001). Many times the chronic eosinophilia is the main reason to suspect of toxocariasis (Magnaval et al., 2001; Pawlovski, 2001; Despommier, 2003). Hepatomegaly, fever and abdominal pain may be found when the compromise is exclusively hepatic (Magnaval et al., 2001). Dry cough, wheezing, bronchospasm, interstitial pneumonitis, and pleural effusion may occur when a lung involvement is present (Roig et al., 1992; Ashwath et al., 2004). Pruritus and eosinophilic urticaria may also present in some patients with dermatological manifestations (Kim et al., 2010). Other manifestations also include arthralgia, vasculitis, pericardial effusion, etc (Pawlovski, 2001; Despommier, 2003).

Ocular toxocariasis is a localized form of toxocariasis and is a result of the ocular invasion by *Toxocara* larvae, causing a series of clinical conditions, including endophthalmitis (Magnaval et al., 2001; Pawlovski, 2001; Despommier, 2003; Smith et al., 2009), which may be confused with a malignant tumor known as retinoblastoma (Minvielle et al., 1999; Magnaval et al., 2001; Despommier, 2003). The parasite is located within the ocular globe and often causes uveitis and retinal granulomas (Dernouchamps et al., 1990), which is confused with other etiologies and which may pass almost unnoticed, since the patient only afflicts progressive decrease in visual acuity (Pawlovski, 2001; Despommier, 2003); some patients present pain or bleeding due to severe intraocular inflammation (Magnaval et al., 2001; Despommier, 2003).

Another localized form of human toxocariasis which has become more important in recent years is the neurotoxocariasis, a clinical entity resulting from the invasion of the brain by *Toxocara* larvae (Finsterer & Auer, 2007). In the brain, *Toxocara* larvae are not encapsulated and the traces of their migration generally include small areas of necrosis and minimal inflammatory infiltration. Therefore, several cases of neurotoxoxariasis are asymptomatic while in others, the symptoms may vary widely. A case-control study on patients with *Toxocara* infection concluded that larval migration in the human brain does not necessarily induce neurological symptoms or signs (Magnaval et al., 1997), but some symptoms such as neurological deficits, focal seizures, generalized behavioral disorders and eosinophilic meningoencephalitis have been reported in different human cases of toxocariasis (Hill et al., 1985; Skerrett & Holland, 1997).

Covert toxocariasis is another form of toxocariasis whose term introduced by Taylor et al. (1987), is less well defined and frequently undiagnosed but it can commonly occur. Covert toxocariasis is characterized by nonspecific signs and symptoms that do not fall into the category of classic visceral larva migrans, ocular toxocariasis or neurotoxocariasis. Covert toxocariasis seems to depend less on a local reaction to the *Toxocara* larvae but is more an organ oriented immunopathological host response to continued stimulation of the host immune system by parasite antigens (Pawlovski, 2001). The clinical expression varies widely and may present as a pulmonary involvement such as asthma, acute bronchitis, pulmonitis with or without a Loeffler syndrome (Feldman & Parker, 1992; Buijs et al., 1997; Inoue et al., 2002), dermatological disorders such as chronic urticaria or eczema (Wolfrom et al., 1995), lymphadenopathy, myositis and a pseudorheumatic syndrome such as arthralgia (le Lauyer et al., 1990; Kraus et al., 1995).

Analysis of the causal relation of *Toxocara* infection with clinically observed symptomatology requires a good clinical knowledge and assessment of laboratory tests including the detection of IgG and IgE specific antibodies, eosinophilia and others (Magnaval et al., 2001; Despommier, 2003). Covert toxocariasis is often confirmed by alleviation or disappearance of specific symptoms and signs after specific anti-helmintic treatment (Magnaval et al., 2001; Pawlovski, 2001; Smith et al., 2009).

Asymptomatic toxocariasis or simply named *Toxocara* infection is often diagnosed by positive serology, occurs mainly in light or old infections and do not require anthelmintic treatment (Huapaya et al., 2009; Smith et al., 2009). Some cases may present mild eosinophilia, but it do not means a hazard for the patient, however, is important to consider this condition, especially in epidemiological studies on this zoonotic disease which are more frequent worldwide (Huapaya et al., 2009).

4. Diagnosis of human toxocariasis

Humans are considered as paratenic hosts within the life cycle of *Toxocara* where the larvae cannot develop into adult worms and, therefore, the parasitological examination of faeces does not contribute to the laboratory diagnosis (Rubinsky-Elefant et al., 2010). The diagnosis of toxocariasis is generally based on clinical signs and symptoms, which are non-specific, epidemiological data (contact with dogs or cats, geophagia, onychophagy, consumption of undercooked or raw meats) and laboratory findings (Chieffi et al., 2009; Despommier, 2003; Magnaval et al., 2001; Watthanakulpanich, 2010).

A definitive diagnosis of human toxocariasis is possible by locating the larvae in infected tissues, using histopathological examination. Tissue biopsy is rarely justified and it is generally insensitive and a time-consuming method (Pawlowski, 2001; Rubinsky-Elefant et al., 2010). Polymerase chain reaction (PCR)-based methods for *Toxocara* identification in clinical and environmental samples have been described (Fogt-Wyrwas et al., 2007; Zhu et al., 2001), but are not widely available. These methods should provide useful tools for the diagnosis and molecular epidemiological investigations of toxocariasis (Li et al. 2007). Parasite antigens can be detected in granulomas by immunohistochemical techniques and are helpful for toxocariasis diagnosis (de Brito et al., 1994; Musso et al., 2007). Medical imaging techniques such as ultrasonography, computed tomography and magnetic resonance imaging have been used to detect granulomatous lesions due to the migration of *Toxocara* larvae in different locations such as liver, nervous system and eye (Degouy et al.,

2001; Magnaval et al., 2001, Watthanakulpanich, 2010). *Toxocara* excreted-secreted products are highly immunogenic and promote a Th2 type immune response, leading to the production of interleukin 4 and 5, and consequently an increase of IgG, IgE antibodies and eosinophilia (Kayes et al., 1980; Del Prete, 1991). In visceral larva migrans, some frequent laboratorial findings are leukocytosis with intense eosinophilia, hypergammaglobulinemia and isohemagglutinin titer elevation (Jacob et al., 1994). However, in ocular toxocariasis, because of larval burden are relatively small, peripheral blood eosinophilia is frequently absent (Glickman & Schantz, 1981).

The diagnosis of ocular toxocariasis is usually based on clinical evaluation with the presence of ocular lesions, such as retinal or peripheral granulomas and endophthalmitis. Anti-*Toxocara* antibody titers are usually higher in visceral larva migrans than in ocular toxocariasis (Elefant et al., 2006). Even low ELISA titres in the serum may be of diagnostic value, but there is no consensus about the cut-off titres for diagnosis (Rubinsky-Elefant et al., 2010).

In covert toxocariasis some patients do not present eosinophilia and symptoms are unspecific (Magnaval et al., 2001). Detection of anti-*Toxocara* antibodies in clinically suspected toxocariasis patients in different samples, such as serum, ocular or cerebrospinal fluid is valuable to establish the diagnosis (Magnaval et al., 2001; Vidal et al., 2003; de Visser et al., 2008; Smith et al., 2009;).

5. Immunoserological techniques for diagnosing human toxocariasis

The limitations of the parasitological techniques to diagnosing human toxocariasis have encouraged numerous researchers to develop practical and accurate immunoassays. Several immunodiagnostic tests have been described, such as intradermal reaction, complement fixation, bentonite flocculation, agar-gel diffusion, indirect hemagglutination, immunofluorescence, radioimmunoassay and immunoenzymatic assays (Glickman & Schantz, 1981). The antigens used in these immunoassays included somatic extracts of adult worms, embryonated eggs, intact or sectioned larvae, and metabolic products of larvae collected *in vitro*.

Nowadays, the excretory-secretory antigens of *T. canis* larvae (TES) are widely used in serodiagnostic tests that are used for both the diagnosis and seroepidemiological studies (Roldán et al., 2010). These antigens are obtained from *in vitro* maintenance of infective larvae and are a mixture of highly immunogenic glycoproteins (Maizels et al., 1993). Since the first description of TES antigens production (De Savigny, 1975), few modifications in the method have been made. Recently, modified protocols for TES antigens production has been reported, increasing the parasite yield up to five fold, improving the larval purity and reducing the execution time of the protocol (Alcântara-Neves et al., 2008; Ponce-Macotela et al., 2011).

The use of validated serodiagnostic tests has provided a good understanding on the prevalence of human exposure to *Toxocara*. Toxocariasis is one of the few human parasitic diseases whose serodiagnosis uses a standardized antigen (Smith et al., 2009). Currently, the best serodiagnostic options are using the ELISA-IgG as a screening test and confirm any positive serum with an immunoblot test. In addition, each positive serum may also be confirmed by using an ELISA-IgE (Magnaval et al., 2001; Smith et al., 2009), as discussed below.

5.1 Enzyme-Linked Immunosorbent Assay

The Enzyme-linked immunosorbent assay (ELISA) test using TES antigens is the most common diagnostic method to detect anti-*Toxocara* IgG antibodies (De Savigny, 1979; Magnaval et al., 2001; Elefant et al., 2006; Smith et al., 2009), but it remains problematic in areas where the polyparasitism is endemic and the possibility of cross-reactions is high, reducing its diagnostic value. False positive results may occur in patients with ascariasis, strongyloidosis, trichinellosis, and fasciolosis (Magnaval et al., 2001; Ishida et al., 2003; Chieffi et al., 2009; Roldán et al., 2009; Smith et al., 2009). In order to reduce the cross-reactivity with other parasites, many authors have proposed previous serum absorption with extracts of a variety of nonhomologous parasites, i.e. pre-incubating serum samples with antigenic extracts of adult stages of *Ascaris suum* (Camargo et al., 1992; Nunes et al., 1997; Elefant et al., 2006), while others use a more comprehensive panel of antigen extracts from nematodes, cestodes and protozoa (Lynch et al., 1988).

The human IgG response elicited by *Toxocara* larvae may persist for many years (Cypess et al., 1977; Elefant et al., 2006) and, therefore, a positive result by ELISA-IgG cannot distinguish between past and current infection (Roldán et al., 2009). Moreover, high levels of anti-*Toxocara* antibodies may be found in preschool children, in comparison with older children or adults living in the same community (Rubinsky-Elefant et al., 2008), suggesting that IgG antibody levels tend to decrease when larvae are no longer viable in tissues.

In human toxocariasis, IgM antibodies are also generated and may be detected in both acute and chronic phases, differing from most of unrelated infections, in which they are transient (Smith, 1993).

Other antibody isotypes, such as IgE, may be detected by ELISA and result more specific than IgG; however, they are less sensitive for the diagnosis of human toxocariasis (Magnaval et al., 1992). In a follow-up of 23 children with visceral toxocariasis, Elefant et al., (2006) found that the levels of IgE antibodies were significantly decreased at one year post-treatment with thiabendazole in comparison with IgG levels which declined only four years post-treatment.

The measurement of the specific IgG avidity by ELISA suggests that it can help in distinguishing between acute and chronic infections (Hubner et al., 2001; Dziemian et al., 2008; Fenow et al., 2008). In the follow-up study after chemotherapy, Elefant et al. (2006) found high-avidity IgG antibodies at the time of the diagnosis, without further increase over the following years.

As an alternative to the ELISA, dot-ELISA has been standardized, presenting comparable sensitivity of standard ELISA. The advantages of the test are related to stability, lower cost and shorter execution time (Camargo et al., 1992; Roldán et al., 2006).

Regarding to the IgG subclasses, IgG2 and IgG3 antibodies yield sensitivities of 98% and 78%, respectively (Watthanakulpanich et al., 2008). On the other hand, the detection of IgG4 antibodies contributes to increase the specificity of the immunoassay (Noordin et al., 2005).

In ocular toxocariasis cases, probably due to the low number of infective larvae, serum anti-*Toxocara* antibodies may be present in very low titres or even undetectable (Sharkey & McKay, 1993; Glickman & Schantz, 1981; Magnaval et al., 2002). However, titers of specific antibodies in intraocular fluids, such as vitreous or aqueous humor, are usually higher than those in serum, suggesting a local antibody production (Biglan et al., 1979; De Visser et al., 2008; Rubinsy-Elefant et al., 2010).

Because of the cross-reactions occurring in populations from tropical areas, some recombinant TES antigens have been expressed and used for the detection of specific IgG (Yamasaki et al., 2000; Wickramasinghe et al., 2008; Mohamad et al., 2009) and IgE antibodies (Norhaida et al., 2008) with promising results. Two of these recombinant antigens named rTES-30 (Yamasaki et al., 2000) and rTES-120 (Fong & Lau., 2004) provide more reliable diagnostic results and may be used for the development of serodiagnostic assays for human toxocariasis.

The detection of circulating *Toxocara* antigens has been reported by a capture enzyme-linked immunoassay using monoclonal antibodies (Robertson et al., 1988; Gillespie et al., 1993). The assay detects a carbohydrate epitope of TES antigens and proved to be useful in confirming acute visceral larva migrans diagnosis. Due to lack of specificity, the test was not recommended to be used alone in diagnosis (Gillespie et al., 1993). A monoclonal antibody to the TES-120 kDa antigen has been described and may be useful for determining both the parasite burden in early infection and the efficacy of chemotherapy (Yokoi et al., 2002).

5.2 Immunoblot assay

The immunoblot or Western blotting assay is a test that combines the high sensitivity of the immunoenzymatic tests with the high resolution of sodium dodecyl sulfate-polyacrylamide gel electrophoresis (SDS-PAGE). This method has been successfully adapted for the confirmatory serodiagnosis of various parasitic diseases, including schistosomiasis, hydatidosis, cysticercosis, taeniasis, fasciolosis and strongyloidosis (as described in Roldán & Espinoza, 2009).

Immunoblot assays based on TES antigens have been proposed as confirmatory tests after screening by ELISA tests (Magnaval et al. 2001; Roldán & Espinoza, 2009). Two clusters of bands have been defined: low molecular weight bands (from 24 to 35 kDa) were reported as highly specific, while the high molecular bands (from 132 to 200 kDa) are unspecific (Magnaval et al., 1991). Morever, Nunes et al. (1997) found that a band between 55 to 66 kDa seems to be the responsible for the cross-reactivity between *T. canis* and *A. suum*.

An immunoblot was standardized for monitoring IgG, IgE and IgA antibodies after-chemotherapy in patients with toxocariasis. IgG antibodies to >205 kDa fractions, IgA to 29–38, 48–54, 81–93 kDa and IgE to 95–121 kDa were suggested as candidates for monitoring the treatment. Further identification of antigen epitopes related to these markers will allow the development of sensitive and specific immunoassays for the diagnosis and therapeutic assessment of toxocariasis (Rubinsky-Elefant et al., 2011).

Nowadays, Immunoblot assay is useful to confirm any positive serum by the ELISA test (where pre-absorption is not carried out) in patients with suspected toxocariasis (Magnaval et al., 1991; Roldán & Espinoza, 2009; Rubinsky-Elefant et al., 2011).

In order to give an idea of how to develop an immunoblot assay using TES antigens to detect specific IgG antibodies, we describe a protocol developed by Roldán & Espinoza (2009), however, we recommend to revise in detail other procedures described by other authors (Magnaval et al., 1991; Nunes et al., 1997; Rubinsky-Elefant et al., 2011).

The TES antigens may be obtained by *in vitro* maintaining larval stages of *T. canis* in RPMI 1640 cell culture medium supplemented with HEPES and glutamine, as described by Bowman et al. (1987). However, it is important to mention that some authors also use the traditional method described by De Savigny (1975), which uses Eagle's minimal essential medium supplemented with HEPES and glutamine (Nunes et al., 1997; Elefant et al., 2006). As a consequence of cultivating the parasite in different kind of culture media, it may generate different antigenic bands at the time of separating the TES antigens by SDS-PAGE.

The TES antigens should be diluted to a final concentration of 200 µg/mL with sample buffer (2.5 mM Tris-HCl, pH 8.0, containing 1% SDS, 50 mM dithiothreitol, 0.4% glycerol and 0.025% bromophenol blue), and then heated at 65°C for 15 min, as recommended by Tsang et al. (1991). In this part, it is important to mention that other authors use Laemmli's sample buffer to dilute the TES antigens.

The TES antigens are separated by SDS-PAGE at a constant voltage of 100V for 15 min (to move the proteins through the stacking gel) and then at 200V (to move the proteins through the resolving gel), until the bromophenol blue reach the end of the gel. Many authors usually have used 10% or 12% resolving polyacrylamide gels (Magnaval et al., 1991; Elefant et al., 2006), but others prefer use gradient resolving gels, such as 5-15% (Nunes et al., 1997; Rubinsky-Elefant et al., 2011) or 4-16% (Roldán & Espinoza, 2009). The relative molecular weight (MW) of the TES antigens may be calculated by using the wide-range molecular weight markers that are commercially available.

The separated TES antigens may be transferred to nitrocellulose sheets (0.2 µm pore size) using an electrotransfer blotting apparatus with a constant current of 2.0 A or a constant voltage of 100V. The time of blotting depends on the model of apparatus and it is very important to follow the instructions described in the manual of each apparatus.

The nitrocellulose sheets containing the TES antigens should be washed for 30 min with 0.01 M phosphate-buffered saline containing 0.3% Tween 20 (PBS-T), and then cut into 3-mm-wide strips and stored at -20°C until use.

These nitrocellulose strips may be incubated with human serum samples diluted at 1:50 in PBS-T containing 5% non-fat milk for 2 hours at room temperature or overnight at 4°C. After this period of incubation, the strips must be washed 3 times for 5 min each with PBS-T and then, the strips must be incubated for 2 hours with an anti-human IgG horseradish peroxidase conjugate diluted 1:1000 in PBS-T. After washing 3 times with PBS-T as above, the strips must be incubated with a freshly prepared substrate solution (15 mg of 3,3' - diaminobenzidine tetrahydrochloride, 30 mL of PBS and 10 µL of 30% hydrogen peroxide). After 5 minutes of incubation, the enzymatic reaction must be stopped by washing the strip with tap water. Positive reactions on the strip are determined by the visualization of defined brown bands judged using the naked eye.

Usually, a total of 9 antigenic bands (24, 28, 30, 35, 56, 67, 117, 136, y 152 kDa) may be detected using this procedure, but the diagnostics bands for the confirmatory serodiagnosis of human toxocariasis are the low molecular weight bands (from 24 to 35 kDa) (figure 1).

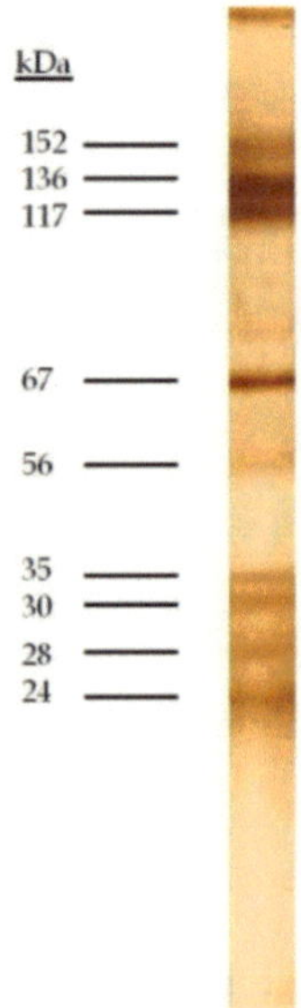

Fig. 1. An immunoblot strip showing the 9 antigenic bands used for the confirmatory serodiagnosis of human toxocariasis.

6. Final considerations

Traditional parasitological diagnostic approaches in toxocariasis, regarding the identification of the larvae, have innumerous limitations. Therefore, laboratory tests are very important to help the clinicians may give a reliable diagnosis. Human toxocariasis has been widely investigated, but many questions about to the diagnosis, effectiveness of chemotherapy, and prognosis remains to be elucidated.

Undoubtedly, the use of the TES antigens in ELISA tests has contributed to improve the immunodiagnosis and to carry out several epidemiological surveys. However, the levels of serum IgG antibodies may remain present for a long time, even in the absence of the disease. When using native unfractionated TES, the probability of cross-reactions may occur in regions where polyparasitism is endemic. In some ocular toxocariasis cases, the serum sample may be repeatable negative without excluding the infection (Smith et al, 2009).

There are some factors that can influence the diagnostic efficiency, such as variation in methods among laboratories, lack of universal units for expressing titers, disagreement in the definition of cut-off lines, differences among surveyed populations and interference of unrelated diseases, such as asthma, in the reactivity of anti-*Toxocara* antibodies (Smith et al. 2009).

Until moment, the ELISA assay is the most widely accepted serodiagnostic test for the detection of anti-*Toxocara* IgG antibodies. Although the ELISA may detect infections by both *T. canis* and *T. cati* (Hotez & Wilkins, 2009), the relative contribution of *T. cati* as etiologic agent of toxocariasis cases has been underestimated (Fisher, 2003). A development of a *T. cati* recombinant antigen would be useful for a better understanding on *T. cati* infection (Smith et al., 2009).

There are many points to be improved in the immunodiagnosis of human toxocariasis, such as the establishment of a standard cut-off value, the definition of true toxocariasis cases and true negative samples.

To establish the final diagnosis of visceral or ocular toxocariasis, clinical signs, symptoms, laboratory data and eosinophil count should be considered (Roldán et al., 2010; Rubinsky-Elefant et al., 2010). On the other hand, the definition of the true negative cases is also complicated and it should be taken in account at the moment of calculating the cut-off values. A positive result in a serological test does not necessarily indicate a causative relationship between *Toxocara* infection and current disease (Pawlowski, 2001). Moreover, in developing countries with a high prevalence of soil-helminth zoonoses is difficult to find true negative serum samples to be used as controls in immunoassays for toxocariasis. Further studies are crucial to improve the sensitivity and specificity of the immunoassays for toxocariasis in order to determine the course of the disease. Tools for distinguish between current or past infection, to improve the diagnosis of ocular toxocariasis, and to define the effectiveness of the therapeutics are needed. Probably, a mixture of recombinant antigens will improve the efficacy of the immunoassays (Mohamad et al., 2009).

7. References

Alcântara-Neves, N.M.; Santos A.B.; Mendonça, L.R.; Figueiredo, C.A.V. & Pontes-de-Carvalho, L. (2008). An improved method to obtain antigen-excreting *Toxocara canis* larvae. *Experimental Parasitology*, Vol.119, No.3, pp. 349–51, ISSN 0014-4894

Araujo, P. (1972). Observacoes pertinentes as priméiras ecdises de larvas de *Ascaris lumbricoides, A. suum* e *Toxocara canis. Revista do Instituto de Medicina Tropical de São Paulo*, Vol.14, No.2, pp. 83-90, ISSN 0036-4665

Ashwath, M.L.; Robinson, D.R. & Katner, H.P. (2004). A presumptive case of toxocariasis associated with eosinophilic pleural effusion: case report and literature review. *American Journal of Tropical Medicine and Hygiene*, Vo.71, No.6, pp. 764, ISSN 0002-9637

Avcioglu, H. & Balkaya, I. (2011). The relationship of public park accessibility to dogs to the presence of *Toxocara* species ova in the soil. Vector Borne and Zoonotic Diseases, Vol.11, No.2, pp. 177-80, ISSN 1530-3667

Biglan, A.W.; Glickman, L.T. & Lobes, L.A. (1979). Serum and vitrous antibody in nematode endophthalmitis. *American Journal of Ophthalmology*, Vol.88, pp. 898-901, ISSN 0002-9394

Buijs, J.; Borsboom, G.; Renting, M.; Hilgersom, W.J.; van Wieringen, J.C.; Jansen, G. & Neijens, J. (1997) Relationship between allergic manifestations and *Toxocara* seropositivity: a cross-sectional study among elementary school children. *European Respiratory Journal* Vol.10, No.7, pp. 1467-75, ISSN 0903-1936

Camargo, E.D.; Nakamura, P.M.; Vaz, A.J.; Silva, M.V.; Chieffi, P.P. & Mello, E.O. (1992). Standardization of DOT-ELISA for the serological diagnosis of toxocariasis and comparison of the assay with ELISA. *Revista do Instituto de Medicina Tropical de São Paulo*, Vol.34, pp. 55-60, ISSN 0036-4665

Chieffi, P.P.; Santos, S.V.; Queiroz, M.L. & Lescano, S.A.Z. (2009). Human toxocariasis: contribution by brazilian researcher. *Revista do Instituto de Medicina Tropical de São Paulo*, Vol.51, No.6, pp. 301-8, ISSN 0036-4665

Cypess, R.H.; Karal, M.H.; Zedian, J.L.; Glickman, L.T. & Gitlin, D. (1977). Larva-specific antibodies in patients with visceral larva migrans. Journal of Infectious Diseases, Vol.135, No.4, pp. 633-40, ISSN 0022-1899

De Brito, T.; Chieffi, P.P.; Peres, B.A.; Santos, R.T.; Gayotto, L.C.C.; Viana, M.R.; Porta, G.P. & Alves, V.A.F. (1994). Immunohistochemical detection of toxocaral antigens in human liver biopsies. *International Journal of Surgical Pathology*, Vol.2, No.2, pp.117-24, ISSN 1066-8969

De Savigny, D.H (1975). In vitro maintenance of *Toxocara canis* larvae and a simple method for production of *Toxocara* ES antigen for use in serodiagnostic tests for visceral larva migrans. *Journal of Parasitology*, Vol.61, No.4, pp.781-2, ISSN 0022-3395

De Savigny, D.H.; Voller A. & Woodruff, A.W. (1979). Toxocariasis: serological diagnosis by enzyme immunoassay. *Journal of Clinical Pathology*, Vol.32, No.3, pp. 284-8, ISSN 0021-9746

De Visser, L.; Rothova, A.; de Boer, J.H.; van Loon, A.M.; Kerkhoff, F.T.; Canninga-van Dijk, M.R.; Weersink, A.Y. & de Groot-Mijnes, J.D. (2008). Diagnosis of ocular toxocariasis by establishing intraocular antibody production. *American Journal of Ophthalmology*, Vol.145, No.2, pp. 369-74, ISSN 0002-9394

Degouy, A.; Menat, C.; Aubin, F., Piarroux, R.; Woronoff-Lemsi & Humbert, P. (2001). La Toxocarose. Presse Médicale, Vol. 30, No.(39-40), pp. 1933-8, ISSN 0755-4982

Del Prete, G.F.; De Carli, M.; Mastromauro C.; Biagiotti, R.; Macchia, D.; Falagiani, P.; Ricci, M. & Romagnani, S. (1991). Purified protein derivative of *Mycobacterium tuberculosis* and excretory-secretory antigen(s) of *Toxocara canis* expand in vitro human T cells with stable and opposite (type 1 T helper or type 2T helper) profile of cytokine production. *Journal of Clinical Investigation*, Vol.88, No.1, pp. 346–50, ISSN 0021-9738

Dernouchamps, J.P.; Verougstraete, C. & Demolder, E. (1990). Ocular toxocariasis: a presumed case of peripheral granuloma. *International ophthalmology*, Vol.14, No.5-6, pp. 383-8, ISSN 0165-5701

Despommier, D. (2003). Toxocariasis: Clinical Aspects, Epidemiology, Medical Ecology and Molecular Aspects. *Clinical Microbiology Reviews*, Vol.16, No.2, pp. 265–72, ISSN 0893-8512

Dubinsky, P. Akao, N.; Reiterová, K. & Konáková, G. (2000). Comparison of the sensitive screening kit with two ELISA sets for detection of anti-*Toxocara* antibodies. *Southeast Asian Journal of Tropical Medicine and Public Health*, Vol.31, No.2, pp. 394-8, ISSN 0125-1562

Dziemian, E.; Zarnowska, H.; Kołodziej-Sobocińska, M. & Machnicka, B (2008). Determination of the relative avidity of the specific IgG antibodies in human toxocariasis. *Parasite Immunology*, Vol.30, No.3, pp. 187-90, ISSN

Elefant, G.R.; Shimizu, S.H.; Sanchez, M.C.A.; Jacob, C.M.A. & Ferreira, A.W. (2006). A serological follow-up of toxocariasis patients after chemotherapy based on the detection of IgG, IgA and IgE antibodies by enzyme-linked immunosorbent assay. *Journal of Clinical and Laboratory Analysis*, Vol.20, No.4, pp. 164-72, ISSN 1098-2825

Feldman, G.J. & Parker, H.W. (1992). Visceral larva migrans associated with the hypereosinophilic syndrome and the onset of severe asthma. *Annals of Internal Medicine*, Vol.116, No.10, pp. 838-40, ISSN 0003-4819

Fenoy S.; Rodero, M.; Pons, E.; Aguila, C. & Cuéllar, C. (2008). Follow-up of antibody avidity in BALB/c mice infected with *Toxocara canis*. *Parasitology*, Vol.135, No.6, pp. 725-33, ISSN 0031-1820

Finsterer, J. & Auer, H. (2007). Neurotoxocarosis. *Revista do Instituto de Medicina Tropical de São Paulo*, Vol.49, No.5, pp. 279-87, ISSN 0036-4665

Fisher, M. (2003). *Toxocara cati*: an underestimated zoonotic agent. *Trends in Parasitology*, Vol.19, No.4, pp.167-70, ISSN 1471-4922

Fogt-Wyrwas, R.; Jarosz, W. & Mizgajska-Wiktor, H. (2007). Utilizing a polymerase chain reaction method for the detection of *Toxocara canis* and *T. cati* eggs in soil. *Journal of Helminthology*, Vol.81, No.1, pp. 75-8, ISSN 0022-149X

Fong, M.Y. & Lau, Y.L. (2004).Recombinant expression of the larval excretory-secretory antigen TES-120 of Toxocara canis in the methylotrophic yeast Pichia pastoris. Parasitology Research, Vol.92, No.2, pp. 173-6, ISSN 0932-0113

Gillespie, S.H.; Bidwell, D.; Voller, A.; Robertson, B.D. & Maizels, R.M. (1993). Diagnosis of human toxocariasis by antigen capture enzyme linked immunosorbent assay. *Journal of Clinical Pathology*, Vol.46, No.6, pp. 551-4, ISSN 0021-9746

Glickman, L.T.; Schantz, P.M. & Cypess, R.H. (1979). Canine and human toxocariasis: review of transmission, pathogenesis, and clinical disease. *Journal of the American Veterinary Medical Association*, Vol.175, No.12, pp. 1265-9, ISSN 0003-1488

Glickman, L.T. & Schantz, P.M. (1981). Epidemiology and pathogenesis of zoonotic toxocariasis. *Epidemiology Reviews*, Vol. 3, pp. 230-50, ISSN 0193-936X

Habluetzel, A.; Traldi, G.; Ruggieri, S.; Attili, A.R.; Scuppa P.; Marchetti, R.; Menghini, G. & Esposito F. (2003). An estimation of *Toxocara canis* prevalence in dogs, environmental egg contamination and risk of human infection in the Marche region of Italy. *Veterinary Parasitology*, Vol.113, No.(3-4), pp. 243-52. ISSN 0304-4017

Hill, I.R.; Denham, D.A. & Scholtz, C.L. (1985). *Toxocara canis* larvae in the brain of a British child. *Transactions of the Royal Society of Tropical Medicine and Hygiene*, Vol.79, No.3, pp. 351-4, ISSN 0035-9203

Holland, C.V.; O'Connor, P.; Taylor, M.R.; Hughes, G.; Girdwood, R.W. & Smith, H. (1991). Families, parks, gardens and toxocariasis. *Scandinavian Journal of Infectious Diseases*, Vol.23, No.2, pp. 225-31, ISSN 0036-5548

Hotez, P.J. & Wilkins, P.P. (2009). Toxocariasis: America's most common neglected infection of poverty and a helminthiasis of global importance? *PLoS Neglected Tropical Diseases*, Vol.3, pp.1-4, ISSN 1935-2735

Huapaya, P.; Espinoza, Y.; Roldán, W. & Jiménez, S. (2009). Toxocariosis humana: ¿problema de salud pública? *Anales de la Facultad de Medicina* (Lima), Vol.70, No.4, pp. 283-90, ISSN 1609-9419

Hubner, J., Uhlikova, M. & Leissova, M. (2001). Diagnosis of the early phase of larval toxocariasis using IgG avidity. *Epidemiologie, Mikrobiologie, Imunologie*, Vol.50, No.2, 67-70, ISSN 1210-7913

Inoue, K.; Inoue, Y.; Arai, T.; Nawa, Y.; Kashiwa, Y.; Yamamoto, S & Sakatani, M. (2002). Chronic eosinophilic pneumonia due to visceral larva migrans. *Internal Medicine*, Vol.41, No.6, pp.478-82, ISSN 0918-2918

Ishida, M.M.I; Rubinsky-Elefant, G.; Ferreira, A.W.; Hoshino-Shimizu, S. & Vaz, A.J. (2003). Helminth antigens (*Taenia solium, Taenia crassiceps, Toxocara canis, Schistosoma mansoni* and *Echinococcus granulosus*) and cross-reactivities in human infections and immunized animals. *Acta Tropica*, Vol.89, No.1, pp. 73–84, ISSN 0001-706X

Jacob, C.M.; Pastorino, A.C.; Peres, B.A.; Mello, E.O.; Okay, Y. & Oselka, G.W. (1994). Clinical and laboratorial features of visceral toxocariasis in infancy. *Revista do Instituto de Medicina Tropical de São Paulo*, Vol.36, No.1, pp. 19-26, ISSN 0036-466

Kayes, SG. (1997) Human toxocariasis and the visceral larva migrans syndrome: correlative immunopathology. Chemical Immunology, Vol.66, pp. 99-124, ISSN 1015-0145.

Kayes , S.G. & Oaks, J.A. (1980). *Toxocara canis*: T lymphocyte function in murine visceral larva migrans and eosinophilia onset. *Experimental Parasitology*, Vol.49, No.1, pp. 47-55, ISSN 0014-4894

Kim, M.H.; Jung, J.W.; Kwon, J.W.; Kim, T.W.; Kim, S.H.; Cho, S.H.; Min, K.U. Kim, Y.Y. & Chang, Y.S. (2010). A case of recurrent toxocariasis presenting with urticaria. *Allergy, asthma & immunology research,* Vo.2, No.4, pp. 267-70, ISSN 2092-7355

Kraus, A.; Valencia, X.; Cabral, A.R. & de la Vega, G. (1995). Visceral larva migrans mimicking rheumatic diseases. *The Journal of Rheumatology.* Vol.22, No.3, pp. 497-500, ISSN 0315-162X

Le Lauyer, B.; Menager, V.; Andebert, C.; Le Ropux, P.; Briguet, M.T. & Boulloche, J. (1990) Inflamatory joint disease as a manifestation of *Toxocara canis* larva migrans. Annales de Pédiatrie, Vol.37, No.7, 445-8, ISSN 0066-2097

Li, M.W.; Lin, R.Q.; Chen, H.H.; Sani, R.A.; Song, H.Q. & Zhu, X.Q. (2007). PCR tools for the verification of the specific identity of ascaridoid nematodes from dogs and cats. Molecular Cell Probes, Vol.21, No.5-6, pp. 349-54, ISSN 0890-8508

Lynch, N.R.; Wilkes, L.K.; Hodgen, A.N. & Turner, K.J. (1988b). Specificity of *Toxocara* ELISA in tropical populations. *Parasite Immunology,* Vol.10, No.3, pp. 323-37, ISSN 0141-9838

Magnaval, J.F.; Fabre, R. ; Maurières, P. ; Charlet, J.P. & De Larrard, B. (1992). Evaluation of an immunoenzymatic assay detecting specific anti-*Toxocara* immunoglobulin E for diagnosis and pos tratament follow-up of human toxocariasis. *Journal of Clinical Microbiology,* Vol.30, No.9, pp. 2269-74, ISSN 0095-1137

Magnaval, J.F.; Fabre, R.; Maurières, P.; Charlet, J.P. & De Larrard, B. (1991). Application of the Western blotting procedure for the immunodiagnosis of human toxocariasis. *Parasitology Research,* Vol.77, No.8, pp. 697-702, ISSN 0932-0113

Magnaval, J.F.; Galindo, V.; Glickman, L.T.; Clanet, M. (1997). Human *Toxocara* infection of the central nervous system and neurological disorders: a case-control study. Parasitology, Vol.115, No.5, pp. 537-43, ISSN 0031-1820

Magnaval, J.F.; Glickman, L.T.; Dorchies, P. & Morassin, B. (2001). Highlights of human toxocariasis. *Korean Journal of Parasitology,* Vol.39, No.1, pp. 1-11, ISSN 0023-4001

Magnaval, J.F.; Malard, L.; Morassin, B. & Fabre, R. (2002). Immunodiagnosis of ocular toxocariasis using Western-blot for the detection of specific anti-*Toxocara* IgG and CAP for the measurement of specific anti-Toxocara IgE. *Journal of Helminthology,* Vol.76, No.4, pp. 335-9, ISSN 0022-149X

Maizels, R.M.; Gems, D.H. & Page, A.P. (1993). Synthesis and secretion of TES antigens from *Toxocara canis* infective larvae. In: *Toxocara* and toxocariasis. Clinical, epidemiological and molecular perspectives, eds. Lewis, J.W. & Maizels, R.M. pp. 141-50. ISBN 0900490306. London: British Society for Parasitology.

Minvielle, M.; Niedfeld M.; Ciarmela M. & Basualdo J. (1999). Toxocariosis causada por *Toxocara canis*: aspectos clínico-epidemiológicos. *Enfermedades Infecciosas y Microbiología Clínica,* Vol.17, No.6, pp. 300-6, ISSN 0213-005X

Mohamad, S.; Azmi, N.C. & Noordin, R. (2009). Development and evaluation of a sensitive and specific assay for diagnosis of human toxocariasis by use of three recombinant antigens (TES-26, TES-30USM, and TES-120). *Journal of Clinical Microbiology,* Vol.47, No.6, pp.1712-7, ISSN 0095-1137

Musso, C.; Castelo, J. S.; Tsanaclis, A. M. & Pereira,F. E. (2007). Prevalence of *Toxocara*-induced liver granulomas, detected by immunohistochemistry, in a series of autopsies at a Children's Reference Hospital in Vitória, ES, Brazil. *Virchows Archives,* Vol.450, No.4, pp. 411–47, ISSN 0945-6317

Noordin, R.; Smith, H.V.; Mohamad, S.; Maizels, R.M. & Fong, M.Y. (2005). Comparison of IgG-ELISA and IgG4-ELISA for *Toxocara* serodiagnosis. *Acta Tropica,* Vol.93, No.1, pp. 57-62, ISSN 0001-706X

Norhaida, A.; Suharni, M.; Liza Sharmani, A.T.; Tuda, J. & Rahmah, N. (2008). rTES-30USM: cloning via assembly PCR, expression, and evaluation of usefulness in the detection of toxocariasis. *Annals of Tropical Medicine and Parasitology*, Vol.102, No.2, pp.151-60, ISSN 0003-4983

Nunes, C.M.; Tundisi, R.N.; Garcia, J.F.; Heinemann, M.B.; Ogassawara, S. & Richtzenhain, L.J. (1997). Cross-reactions between *Toxocara canis* and *Ascaris suum* in the diagnosis of visceral larva migrans by Western-blotting technique. *Revista do Instituto de Medicina Tropical de São Paulo*, Vol.39, No.5, pp.253–56, ISSN 0036-466

O'Lorcain, P. (1995). The effects of freezing on the viability of *Toxocara canis* and *T. cati* embryonated eggs. *Journal of Helminthology*, Vol.69, No.2, pp. 169-71, ISSN 0022-149X

Overgaauw, P.A. (1997). Aspects of *Toxocara* epidemiology: toxocarosis in dogs and cats. *Critical reviews in Microbiology*, Vol.23, No.3, pp. 233-51, ISSN 1040-841X

Pawlowski, Z. (2001). Toxocariasis in humans: clinical expression and treatment dilemma. *Journal of Helminthology*, Vol.75, No.4, pp. 299-305, ISSN 0022-149X

Ponce-Macotela, M.; Rodríguez-Caballero, A.; Peralta-Abarca, G.E. & Martínez-Gordillo, M.N. (2011). A simplified method for hatching and isolating *Toxocara canis* larvae to facilitate excretory–secretory antigen collection in vitro. *Veterinary Parasitology*, Vol. 175, No. 3-4, pp. 382–385, ISSN 0304-4017

Robertson, B.D.; Burkot, T.R.; Gillespie, S.H.; Kennedy, M.W.; Wanbai, F. & Maizels, R.M. (1988). Detection of circulating parasite antigen and specific antibody in *Toxocara canis* infections. *Clinical and Experimental Immunology*, Vol.74, No.2, pp. 236-241, ISSN 0009-9104

Roig, J.; Romeu, J.; Riera, C.; Texido, A.; Domingo, C. & Morera, J. (1992). Acute eosinophilic pneumonia due to toxocariasis with bronchoalveolar lavage findings. *Chest*, Vol.102, No.1, pp. 294-96, ISSN 0012-3692

Roldán, W.; Cornejo, W. & Espinoza, Y. (2006). Evaluation of the dot enzyme-linked immunosorbent assay in comparison with standard ELISA for the immunodiagnosis of human toxocariasis. *Memórias do Instituto Oswaldo Cruz*, Vol.101, No.1, pp. 71-74, ISSN 0074-0276

Roldán, W.H. & Espinoza, Y.A. (2009). Evaluation of an enzyme-linked immunoelectrotransfer blot test for the confirmatory serodiagnosis of human toxocariasis. *Memórias do Instituto Oswaldo Cruz*, Vol.104, No.3, pp. 411-18, ISSN 0074-0276

Roldán, W.H.; Espinoza, Y.A.; Huapaya, P.E. & Jiménez, S. (2010). Diagnóstico de la toxocarosis humana. *Revista Peruana de Medicina Experimental y Salud Publica*, Vol.27, No.4, pp. 613-20, ISSN 1726-4634

Rubinsky-Elefant, G.; Hirata, C.E.; Yamamoto, J.H. & Ferreira, M.U. (2010). Human toxocariasis: diagnosis, worldwide seroprevalences and clinical expression of the systemic and ocular forms. *Annals of Tropical Medicine & Parasitology*, Vol.104, No.1, pp. 3-23, ISSN 0003-4983

Rubinsky-Elefant, G.; Hoshino-Shimizu, S.; Jacob, C.M.A.; Sanchez, M.C.A. & Ferreira, A.W. (2011). Potential immunological markers for diagnosis and therapeutic assessment of toxocariasis. *Revista do Instituto de Medicina Tropical de São Paulo*, Vol.53, No.2, pp. 61-5, ISSN 0036-4665

Schantz, P.M. & Glickman, L.T. (1978). Toxocaral visceral larva migrans. New England Journal of Medicine, Vol.298, No.8, pp. 436-9. ISSN 0028-4793

Sharkey, J.A. & McKay, P.S. (1993). Ocular toxocariasis in a patient with repeatedly negative ELISA titre to *Toxocara canis*. *British Journal of Ophthalmology*, Vol.77, No.4, pp. 253-4, ISSN 0007-1161

Skerrett, H. & Holland, C.V. (1997). Variation in the larval recovery of *Toxocara canis* from the murine brain: implications for behavioural studies. *Journal of helminthology.* Vol.71, No.3, pp.253-5, ISSN 0022-149X

Smith, H.; Holland, C.; Taylor, M.; Magnaval, J-F.; Schantz, P. & Maizel, R. (2009). How common is human toxocariasis? Towards standardizing our knowledge. *Trends in Parasitology*, Vol.25, No.4, pp. 182-8, ISSN 1471-4922

Sugane, K. & Oshima, T. (1984). Interrelationship of eosinophilia and IgE antibody production to larval ES antigen in *Toxocara canis* infected mice. *Parasite Immunology*, Vol.6, No.5, pp. 409-20, ISSN 0141-9838

Taylor, M.R.; Keane, C.T.; O'Connor, P.; Girdwood, R.W. & Smith, H. (1987). Clinical features of covert toxocariasis. *Scandinavian Journal of Infectious Diseases*, Vol.19, No.6, pp. 693-6, ISSN 0036-5548

Taylor, M.R.; Keane, C.T.; O'Connor, P.; Mulvihill, E. & Holland, C. (1988). The expanded spectrum of toxocaral disease. Lancet, Vol.1, No.8587, pp. 692-5, ISSN 0140-6736

Uga, S.; Minami, T. & Nagata, K. (1996). Defecation habits of cats and dogs and contamination by *Toxocara* eggs in public park sandpits. *American Journal of Tropical Medicine and Hygiene*, Vol.54, No.2, pp. 122-6, ISSN 0002-9637

Vidal, J.E.; Sztajnbok, J. & Seguro, A.C. (2003). Eosinophilic meningoencephalitis due to *Toxocara canis*: case report and review of the literature. *American Journal of Tropical Medicine and Hygiene*, Vol.69, No.3, pp. 341–3, ISSN 0002-9637

Watthanakulpanich, D. (2010). Diagnostic trends of human toxocariasis. *Journal of Tropical Medicine and Parasitology*, Vol.33, pp. 44-52, ISSN 0125-4987

Watthanakulpanich, D.; Smith, H.V.; Hobbs, G.; Whalley, A.J. & Billington, D. (2008). Application of *Toxocara canis* excretory-secretory antigens and IgG subclass antibodies (IgG1-4) in serodiagnostic assays of human toxocariasis. *Acta Tropica*, Vol.106, No.2, pp. 90-5, ISSN 0001-706X

Wickramasinghe, S.; Yatawara, L.; Nagataki, M.; Takamoto, M.; Watanabe, Y.; Rajapakse, R.P.; Uda, K., Suzuki, T. & Agatsuma, T. (2008). Development of a highly sensitive IgG-ELISA based on recombinant arginine kinase of *Toxocara canis* for serodiagnosis of visceral larva migrans in the murine model. *Parasitology Research*, Vol.103, No.4, pp.853-8, ISSN 0932-0113

Wolfrom, E.; Chêne, G.; Boisseau, H.; Beylot, C.; Géniaux, M. & Taïeb, A. (1995). Chronic urticaria and *Toxocara canis*. Lancet, Vol.345, No.8943, pp. 196, ISSN 0140-6736

Yamasaki, H.; Araki, K.; Lim, P.K.C.; Zasmy, N.; Mak, J.W.; Taib, R. & Aoki, T. (2000). Development of a highly specific recombinant *Toxocara canis* second-stage larva excretory-secretory antigen for immunodiagnosis of human toxocariasis. *Journal of Clinical Microbiology*, Vol. 38, No.4, pp. 1409-13, ISSN 0095-1137

Yokoi, K.; Kobayashi, F.; Sakai, J.; Usui, M. & Tsuji, M. (2002). Sandwich ELISA detection of excretory-secretory antigens of *Toxocara canis* larvae using a specific monoclonal antibody. *Southeast Asian Journal of Tropical Medicine and Public Health*, Vol. 33, No.1, pp. 33-7, ISSN 0125-1562

Zhu, X.Q.; Gasser, R.B.; Chilton, N.B. & Jacobs, D.E. (2001). Molecular approaches for studying ascaridoid nematodes with zoonotic potential, with an emphasis on *Toxocara* species. *Journal of Helminthology*, Vol.75, No.2, pp. 101-8, ISSN 0022-149X

8

Recent Advances in the Immunology and Serological Diagnosis of Echinococcosis

Wenbao Zhang[1,2,*], Jun Li[1,2], Renyong Lin[1], Hao Wen[1] and Donald P. McManus[2]
[1]*State Key Laboratory Breeding Base of Xinjiang Major Diseases Research, Clinical Medicine Institute, First Affiliated Hospital of Xinjiang Medical University, Urumqi,*
[2]*Molecular Parasitology Laboratory, Australian Centre for International and Tropical Health and Nutrition, The Queensland Institute of Medical Research and The University of Queensland, Brisbane,*
[1]*China*
[2]*Australia*

1. Introduction

Echinococcosis is a near-cosmopolitan zoonosis caused by tapeworms (cestodes) belonging to the family Taeniidae and the genus *Echinococcus*. This parasitic disease is very common but largely neglected. The two major species of medical and public health importance are *Echinococcus granulosus* (*Eg*) and *E. multilocularis* (*Em*), which cause cystic echinococcosis (CE) and alveolar echinococcosis (AE), respectively. Globally, CE is responsible for most of the burden of echinococcosis (Budke, 2006), although AE is re-emerging with increasing frequency in Europe (Deplazes, 2006; Eckert *et al.*, 2000; Romig, 2009; Hegglin *et al.*, 2008).

There are 4 million people infected and more than 100 million at risk of infection including many in the EU countries (Craig and Larrieu, 2006; Craig *et al.*, 2007; McManus *et al.*, 2003). In the endemic regions, human incidence rates can reach more than 50 per 100 000 person/year and prevalence as high as 5-10% may occur, as in parts of Peru, Argentina, east Africa and central Asia (Altintas, 2003; Craig *et al.*, 2007; Moro *et al.*, 1997). In China, there are 60 million people at risk (Ito *et al.*, 2003b) with 550,000 CE patients having visible hydatid cysts by ultrasound (Collaboration projects, 2005; Li *et al.*, 2005) and > 100 million animals infected(Chi *et al.*, 1989).

2. Life-cycle and Echinococcosis

The complex life cycle of *Echinococcus* involves two hosts (Fig 1); a definitive host and an intermediate host. Definitive hosts are carnivores such as dogs, wolves and foxes. Sexual maturity of adult *E. granulosus* occurs in the host small intestine within 4 to 5 weeks of

* Corresponding Author

ingesting offal containing viable protoscoleces. Gravid proglottids or released eggs are shed in the feces.

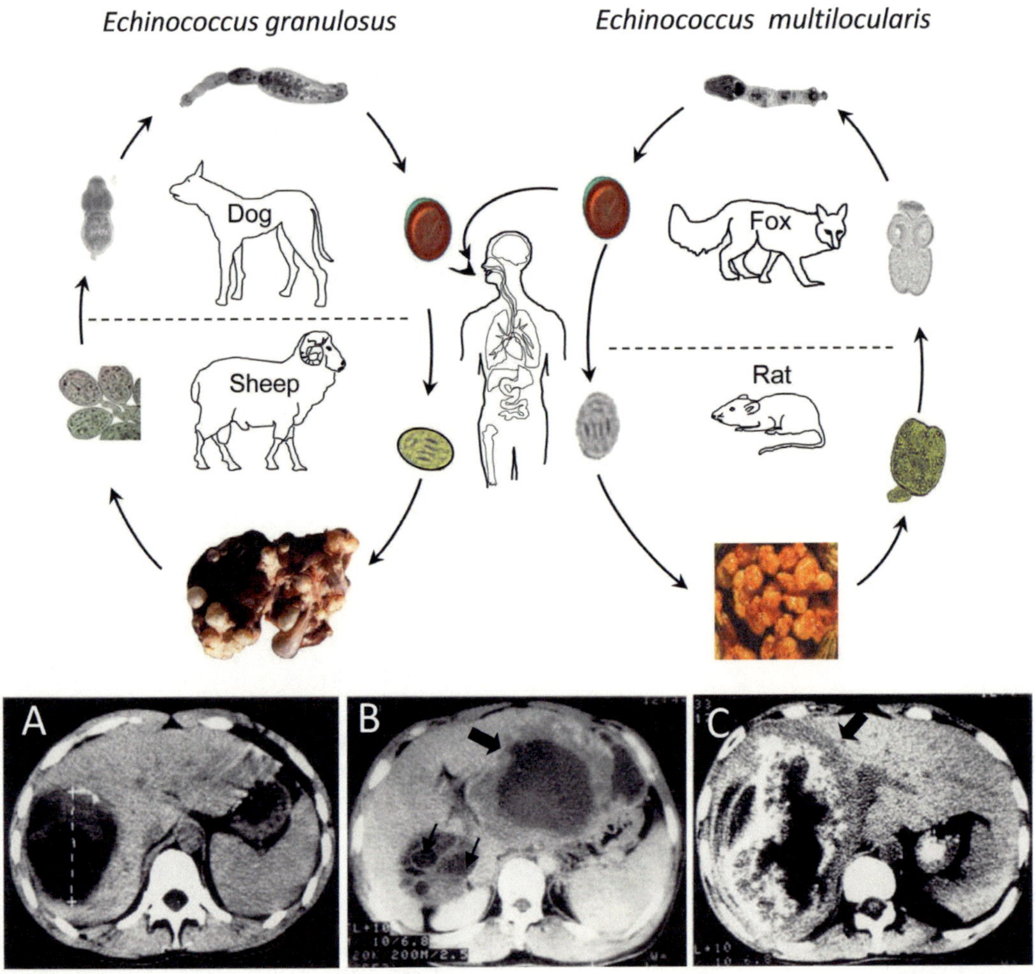

Fig. 1. Life cycle of *Echinococcus* (upper panel) and hepatic echinococcosis scanned by computed axial tomography (CT) (lower panels). A, Cystic echinococcosis (CE) due to *E. granulosus*. B, a patient infected with both CE (daughter cysts are marked with small arrowheads) and alveolar echinococcosis (AE, large arrowhead). C, AE due to *E. multilocularis* infection (arrowhead).

Intermediate hosts are herbivores such as sheep, horses, cattle, pigs, goats, camels, moose, kangaroos and wallabies. Humans are accidental hosts and generally play no part in transmission. Intermediate hosts and humans become infected by ingesting eggs of the parasites, which are released in the faeces of the definitive hosts. The eggs hatch in the gastrointestinal tract and become activated larvae (oncospheres) which penetrate the intestinal wall and enter the bloodstream, eventually locating in internal organs, where they develop into hydatid cysts. Hydatid cysts of *E. granulosus* develop in internal organs of intermediate hosts and humans as fluid-filled bladders (Figure 1A). The cysts can be located in almost all organs, with about 70% of cysts in the liver, 20% in the lungs, with the remainder involving other organs such as the kidney, spleen, brain, heart and bone.

A typical cyst of *E. granulosus* consists of two parasite-derived layers; an inner nucleated germinal layer and an outer acellular laminated layer surrounded by a host-produced fibrous capsule. Brood capsules and protoscoleces bud off from the germinal membrane.

The alveolar cyst or metacestode of *E. multilocularis* develops differently to that of *E. granulosus,* being a complex tumor-like multivesicular, infiltrating structure consisting of numerous small vesicles embedded in stroma of connective tissue (Fig 1B and C). The larval mass usually contains a semisolid matrix, rather than fluid, with granulomatous infiltration of mononuclear cells around the parasitic vesicles, a hallmark of AE, culminating in irreversible fibrosis. Adult worm infections of *E. multilocularis* occur mainly in red and arctic foxes, although dogs and cats (rarely) can also act as definitive hosts. Small mammals (usually microtine and arvicolid rodents) act as intermediate hosts (Fig 1).

The chronic disease of CE is characterized in humans and domestic and wild ungulates by long term growth of metacestode (hydatid) cysts in the internal organs of intermediate hosts. Clinical manifestations are mild in the early stages of infection, and normally remain asymptomatic for a long period, but the host does produce detectable humoral and cellular responses against the infection, while the parasite has evolved highly effective evasive strategies to aid in long term survival. Immunity to *E. granulosus* infection is typical of a chronic infection and the host responses are pivotal for developing laboratory-based diagnostic procedures.

The proliferative larval stages of *E. granulosus* and *E. multilocularis* can 'leak" out of a ruptured cyst (*E. granulosus*) or metastisize (*E. multilocularis*) to another organ or tissue naturally producing a condition known as secondary CE or AE, respectively. This also allows the parasites to be passaged serially from one intermediate host to another by intraperitoneal implantation of the larvae, simplifying the technical difficulties and danger associated with cyclic passage through both definitive and intermediate hosts.

CE and AE are both serious diseases, the latter especially so, with a poor prognosis if careful clinical management is not carried out. In the later stages of echinococcosis, as the disease progresses, the parasite may physically damage tissues and organs which can become dysfunctional and can be fatal, especially in AE, when the parasite destroys the liver parenchyma, bile ducts and blood vessels resulting in biliary obstruction and portal hypertension. In most late-stage cases a necrotic cavity, containing viscous fluid, may form in the liver.

3. Host immune responses against infection

Immune responses play an important role in the host-parasite interplay in echinococcosis. The mammalian host produces immune responses to reject and/or limit the growth of the parasite, whereas, the parasite produces molecules to avoid these immune attacks. One phenomenon of the infection is self-cure, which is commonly observed in sheep (Zhang and Zhao, 1992; Cabrera *et al.*, 2003) and also occurs in humans in hyper-endemic areas (Wang *et al.*, 2006; Moro *et al.*, 2005; Macpherson *et al.*, 2004). Indeed, more than 70% of cysts surgically removed from a large cohort of Chinese patients were shown to be inactive and calcified (Peng, XY, personal communication), indicating that the number of human self-cure cases can be substantial. However, details of this important, likely immunologically-based process, remain limited. In addition, some intermediate hosts such as cattle produce a high percentage - >90% - of cysts that are infertile in that they do not contain protoscoleces, the developmental form of the parasite infective to the definitive host (Fig. 1), with host species-specific differences in immunity probably the key factor (Zhang *et al.*, 2003a). Similarly in AE, some patients with calcified lesions (Gottstein and Felleisen, 1995) are likely due to self-cure.

This self-cure phenomenon raises the possibility that protective immune responses against parasite growth and dissemination may exist. However, little is known about the determinants which may restrain metacestode survival and proliferation, or eliminate *Echincococcus* infection.

Although the data are limited, there is, nevertheless, clear evidence, from experiments with animals challenged with *E. granulosus/E. multilocularis* eggs or oncospheres that infected hosts produce significant immune responses, including antibody and T cell responses generated by lymphocytes. Understanding the mechanisms whereby these immune responses are produced, particularly the role of protective antibodies against the oncosphere, has been of fundamental importance in developing highly effective recombinant vaccines against both *E. granulosus* and *E. multilocularis*.

3.1 Antibody responses

The earliest immunoglobin (Ig) G response to *E. granulosus* hydatid cyst fluid and oncospheral antigens appears after 2 and 11 weeks, respectively, in mice and sheep challenged with eggs or oncospheres of *E. granulosus* (Zhang *et al.*, 2003b; Yong *et al.*, 1984). Anti-oncospheral antibodies play a major role in parasite killing and are central to the protective immune response against *E. granulosus* (Read *et al.*, 2009). In the chronic phase of CE, elevated antibody levels, particularly IgG, IgM and IgE, occur in humans (Khabiri *et al.*, 2006; Daeki *et al.*, 2000; Pinon *et al.*, 1987; Craig, 1986; Dessaint *et al.*, 1975) (Fig. 2), with IgG1 and IgG4 being predominant (Daeki *et al.*, 2000; Sterla *et al.*, 1999; Wen and Craig, 1994). In murine models of AE infection, IgG and IgM were significantly increased after 9 weeks post-infection (p.i) with eggs (Matsumoto *et al.*, 2010). Antibody responses to protoscolex antigens are relatively weak and delayed in the early stage of *E. multilocularis* infection in mice, but are increased later (Bauder *et al.*, 1999; Matsumoto *et al.*, 1998); IgG1 and IgG3 levels increase significantly at 8 weeks p.i, and remain elevated thereafter (Li *et al.*, 2003a).

Antibody production is a pre-requisite for the development of serodiagnostic tests, but 30-40% of patients are antibody-negative for CE. In many of these patients, however, varying levels of circulating antigens (CAg) and circulating immune complexes (CIC) are measurable (Craig, 1993). This phenomenon suggests that B cell activity and proliferation may be regulated and inhibited by *E. granulosus* antigens. It is not known whether these antigens directly target B cells or via T cell regulatory mechanisms. One study showed that after infection, CD4-knockout mice and C57Bl/6 mice had similar titres of specific antibodies, indicating that antibody production may be T cell-independent in early infection (Baz *et al.*, 2008).

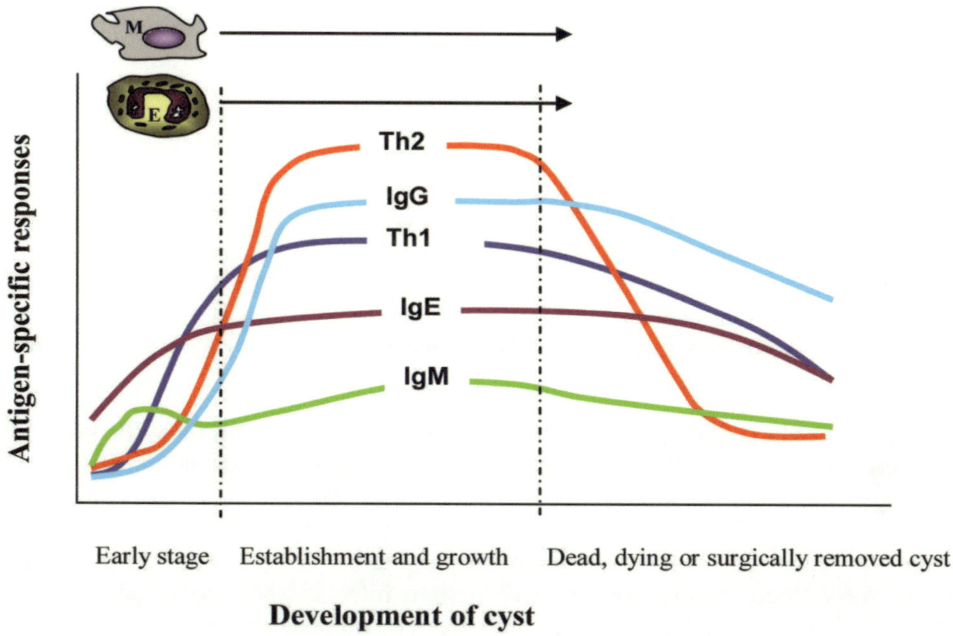

Fig. 2. Immune responses during the development of a hydatid cyst of *E. granulosus* in the intermediate host. In the early stage of infection, the oncosphere is transported to a host organ such as the liver or lung where it develops into a hydatid cyst. The immature cyst has to overcome host, mainly cell-mediated, immune responses, especially the infiltration of macrophages and eosinophils and low level polarized Th1 responses. About 8-10 weeks post-infection in mice, cyst growth is maintained and complex echinococcal antigens are released from the cyst. These antigens stimulate complex immune responses. These include polarized Th2 responses, balanced with Th1 responses. At this time, the parasite produces significant quantities of antigens that help to modulate the immune response, which may benefit both host and parasite; IgG, especially IgG1 and IgG4, IgE and IgM levels are elevated. When the cyst is dead, dying or surgically removed, the Th2 responses drop rapidly, whereas the Th1 responses drop slowly then becoming polarized. IgG can be maintained in the human host for many years after the cyst is surgically removed. Once an infected patient has relapsed, the Th2 responses recover very quickly, while other responses are elevated slowly. M, macrophage; E, eosinophil.

In addition, antibody responses may indicate the infectious status (Li *et al.*, 2010; Delunardo *et al.*, 2010; Reiter-Owona *et al.*, 2009; Ben Nouir *et al.*, 2008; Ortona *et al.*, 2005). A survey of 246 CE patients showed that *E. granulosus* antigen B (AgB) specific antibody was elevated in a significantly greater proportion (87.3%) of subjects with active or transitional stage cysts (CE1, CE2, or CE3), compared with 54.8% of other patients with inactive or early stage cysts (CL, CE4 or CE5). Furthermore, AgB-specific antibody was detected in 95.6% of CE2 cases, which was statistically higher than that (73.7%) in CE1 patients (Li *et al.*, 2010). Results from 173 AE patients showed that serum antibody levels against Em18 were significantly correlated with the disease phase (Li *et al.*, 2010).

A survey of 861 children in China showed that serological tests can also be as an indicator of *Echinococcus* transmission; this study predicated the transmission of echinococcosis due to changes in the ecology and socio-geography in and around endemic communities (Yang *et al.*, 2008).

3.2 T cell responses

During the early stages of an echinococcal infection, there is a marked activation of cell-mediated immunity including cellular inflammatory responses and pathological changes (Zhang *et al.*, 2003a; Zhang *et al.*, 2008b). Cellular infiltration of eosinophils, neutrophils, macrophages, and fibrocytes occurs in humans (Magambo *et al.*, 1995; Peng *et al.*, 2006) and sheep (Petrova, 1968) infections. However, this generally does not result in a severe inflammatory response and aged cysts tend to become surrounded by a fibrous layer that separates the laminated cystic layer from host tissue.

Early Th1 polarized cytokine production, which can kill the metacestode at the initial stages of development (Vuitton, 2003), then shifts to a predominant Th2 cytokine response in the later, chronic stage, and is characteristic of *E. granulosus* and *E. multilocularis* infection (Fig. 2). Very little is known of cytokine production in the early phases of a primary (oral challenge with eggs) *E. granulosus* infection, although both Th1 and Th2 cytokine levels are low in the early stages of a primary *E. multilocularis* infection, but are raised subsequently (Bauder *et al.*, 1999). As well, it is thought the Th2 cytokines are responsible for inhibition of parasite killing because of the anti-inflammatory action of interleukin-10 (IL-10) (Bauder *et al.*, 1999; Vuitton, 2003). The Th2-type cytokines profile in abortive AE patients was opposite to those in progressive patients, with IL -10 and IL-5 associated with the progression of disease (Godot *et al.*, 2000). However, secondary *E. multilocularis* infection in a mouse model showed that Th1 cytokines play a role in resistance of parasite growth (Emery *et al.*, 1997).

Patients with chronic CE generate both Th1 and Th2 responses (Baz *et al.*, 2006). Given the recent advances in understanding the immunoregulatory capabilities of helminthic infections, it has been suggested that Th2 responses play a crucial role in chronic helminthiasis (Allen and Maizels, 2011). However, a remarkable feature of chronic CE infection is the coexistence of interferon-gamma (IFN-γ), IL-4 and IL-10 at high levels in human echinococcosis (Mezioug and Touil-Boukoffa, 2009). It is unclear why hydatid infection can induce high levels of both Th1 and Th2 cytokines (Rigano *et al.*, 1995a) since they usually down-regulate each other (Pearce and MacDonald, 2002). Antigen and the amount of antigens released may play key roles. For instance, *E. granulosus* AgB skewed Th1/Th2 cytokine ratios towards a preferentially immunopathology-associated Th2 polarization, predominantly in patients with progressive disease (Rigano *et al.*, 2001).

Liver pathology in AE is characterized by the presence of a huge granulomatous infiltrate of mononuclear cells involving mainly macrophages, myofibroblasts and T lymphocytes (Harraga *et al.*, 2003; Vuitton *et al.*, 1989). In the progressive forms of the disease, the T cell infiltrate within the periparasitic granuloma is mainly composed of CD8 T lymphocytes (Bresson-Hadni *et al.*, 1990).

A hallmark of chronic *Echinococcus* infection is the presence of high levels of IL–10 (Zhang *et al.*, 2008a; Vuitton, 2003), a cytokine typically associated with immunoregulation of effector responses (Moore *et al.*, 2001). The role of IL-10 in chronic infection largely remains unclear, although one report showed that IL-10 may impair the Th1 protective response and allow the parasite to survive in hydatid patients (Moore *et al.*, 2001). By inducing the host to produce high levels of IL-10, *E. multilocularis* appears able to modulate the immune response so that the T cells infiltrating the periparasitic granuloma cannot participate in the effector phase of the cellular immune response (Zhang *et al.*, 2008a; Vuitton, 2003). The interaction of the *Echinococcus* organisms with their mammalian hosts may provide a highly suitable model to address some of the fundamental questions remaining such as the molecular basis underpinning the different effects of IL-10 on different cell types; the mechanisms of regulation of IL-10 production; the inhibitory role of IL-10 on monocyte/macrophage and CD4 T cell function; its involvement in stimulating the development of B cells and CD8 T cells; and its role in the differentiation and function of T regulatory cells.

In addition, the production of subgroups of chemokines (CC and CXC) associated with inflammation (MIP-1 alpha(macrophage inflammatory protein 1 alpha)/CCL3, MIP-1 beta/CCL4, RANTES (regulated upon activation, normally T-cell expressed and secreted)/CCL5 and GRO-alpha (growth-regulated oncogene-alpha)/CXCL1) in peripheral blood mononuclear cells stimulated with Em antigens *in vitro* was constitutively larger in AE patients than in controls(Kocherscheidt *et al.*, 2008). However, in patients, Em metacestodes suppressed cellular chemokine production, and this may constitute an immune escape mechanism which reduces inflammatory host responses, prevents tissue destruction and organ damage, but may also facilitate parasite persistence (Kocherscheidt *et al.*, 2008).

It is not known whether the significant cellular infiltration of macrophages and neutrophils occurring as the parasite develops results from the innate immune mechanisms of the host and the release of chemotactic substances by the parasite or whether it is dependent on Th0/Thl cytokines. A large number of CD4(+) T lymphocytes are present in AE patients with aborted or dead lesions, whereas patients with active parasites display a significant increase in activation of predominantly CD8(+) T cells (Manfras *et al.*, 2002) indicating that CD4(+) T cells may play a role in the killing mechanism. This is supported by experiments undertaken with genetically modified mice (Dai *et al.*, 2001). Conversely, *E. multilocularis* is able to survive and persist in its host indefinitely for long periods of time. In fact, the murine immune response fails to clear infection even when presented with the lowest possible infection dose by injection with a single parasite vesicle (Gottstein *et al.*, 2002).

3.3 Correlation of cytokines with antibody production

It is noteworthy that the increased production of IL-4 and IL-10 in hydatid patients (Bayraktar *et al.*, 2005) corresponds with high levels of IgE and IgG4 (Rigano *et al.*, 1995b), suggesting regulation by IL-4 of IgE and IgG4 responses (Rigano *et al.*, 2001; Rigano *et al.*, 1995b; King and Nutman, 1993). Patients with a primary infection have higher levels of IL-2, IFN-γ and IL-5. The effect of IL-5 on human B cells is controversial (Clutterbuck *et al.*, 1989), but a significant correlation between IL-5 production and IgE/IgG4 expression has been found in hydatid patients (Rigano *et al.*, 1996), indicating that IL-5 is associated with the regulation of specific IgE/IgG4 expression. When CE cysts grow, IgG1 and IgG4 levels are elevated, whereas the concentrations of specific IgG1 and IgG4 decline in cases characterized by cyst infiltration or calcification. This indicates that the IgG4 antibody response is also associated with cystic development, growth and disease progression, whereas the IgG1, IgG2 and IgG3 responses occur predominantly when cysts become infiltrated or are destroyed by the host (Daeki *et al.*, 2000).

3.4 T cell responses and treatment

The polarized T cell responses in echinococcosis have been shown to be modulated by the developmental status of the hydatid cyst, as shown by experiments with T-cell lines generated from patients with active, transitional and inactive hydatid cysts and stimulated with sheep hydatid fluid antigens. It is likely due to the antigens containing distinct epitopes for each T-cell subset as a single recombinant protein can stimulate both types of response (Zhang *et al.*, 2003a). T-cell lines from a patient with an inactive cyst had a Th1 profile, while T-cell lines derived from patients with active and transitional hydatid cysts had mixed Th1/Th2 and Th0 clones (Rigano *et al.*, 2004), indicating that Th1 lymphocytes contribute significantly to the inactive stage of hydatid disease, with Th2 lymphocytes being more important in the active and transitional stages. When CE patients were drug-treated with albendazole/mebendazole, a Th1 cytokine profile, rather than a Th2 profile, typically dominated, indicating that Th1 responses have a role in the process of cyst degeneration (Rigano *et al.*, 1995b). An increased Th1-type cytokine IFN-γ response has been suggested as a marker for monitoring AE patient treatment (Dvoroznakova *et al.*, 2004), whereas as measurement of serum IL-4 may be a useful marker for the follow up of patients with CE (Rigano *et al.*, 1999b).

One aspect that is likely to be important in the control of such immunological mechanisms is the influence of CD4+ T-helper lymphocytes as they may impact on treatment of echinococcosis (Vuitton, 2004). As indicated earlier, self-cure is a common feature of CE infection in sheep (Zhang and Zhao, 1992; Cabrera *et al.*, 2003), and it most likely also happens in human populations in hyper-endemic areas as patients with calcified cysts are often reported (Moro *et al.*, 2005; Macpherson *et al.*, 2004). Cytokines are likely to play a key role in the process of self-cure and this is an important area that needs further research.

Both *in vitro* and *in vivo* studies have shown that high levels of the Th1 cytokine IFN-γ were found in patients who responded to chemotherapy, whereas high levels of Th2 cytokines l (IL-4 and IL-10) occurred in patients who did not (Rigano *et al.*, 1999b; Rigano *et al.*, 1999a; Rigano *et al.*, 1995b; Rigano *et al.*, 1995a).

3.5 Dendritc cells

Some recent studies have focused on dendritic cells (DC) and their regulation on other immune responses in CE. *E. granulosus* antigens influence maturation and differentiation of DC stimulated with lipopolysaccharide (LPS) (Kanan and Chain, 2006). This includes down-modulation of CD1a expression and up-regulation of CD86 expression, a lower percentage of CD83(+) cells being present, and down-regulation of interleukin-12p70 (IL-12p70) and TNF alpha (Rigano *et al.*, 2007). In addition, hydatid cyst fluid (HCF) modulates the transition of human monocytes to DC, impairs secretion of IL-12, IL-6 or PGE2 in response to LPS stimulation, and modulates the phenotype of cells generated during culture, resulting in increased CD14 expression (Kanan and Chain, 2006). AgB has been shown to induce IL-1 receptor-associated kinase phosphorylation and activate nuclear factor-kappa B, suggesting that Toll-like receptors could participate in *E. granulosus*-stimulated DC maturation (Rigano *et al.*, 2007).

E. multilocularis infection in mice induced DC expressing high levels TGF and very low levels of IL-10 and IL-12, and the expression of the surface markers CD80, CD86 and CD40 was down-regulated (Mejri *et al.*, 2011a; Mejri *et al.*, 2011b). However, the higher level of IL-4 than IFN-γ/IL-2 mRNA-expression in AE-CD4+ pT cells indicated DC play a role in the generation of a regulatory immune response (Mejri *et al.*, 2011a).

Different *E. multilocularis* antigens have been shown to stimulate different expression profiles of DC. Em14-3-3-antigen induced CD80, CD86 and MHC class II surface expression, but Em2(G11) failed to do so. Similarly, LPS and Em14-3-3 yielded elevated IL-12, TNF-I+/- and IL-10 expression levels, while Em2(G11) did not. The proliferation of bone marrow DC isolated from AE-diseased mice was abrogated (Margos *et al.*, 2011), indicating the *E. multilocularis* infection inhibited T cell responses.

3.6 Regulatory T cells

Chronic *Echinococcus* infection results in the suppression of host immune responses, allowing long-term parasite survival and restricting pathology. Current theories suggest that regulatory T cells (Treg) play an important role in this regulation. However, the mechanism of Treg induction during *Echinococcus* infection is still unknown, although several studies have focused on this area.

A subpopulation of regulatory CD4+ CD25+ T cells isolated from *E. multilocularis*-infected mice reduced ConA-driven proliferation of CD4+ pT cells. The high expression levels of Foxp3 mRNA by CD4+ and CD8+ peritoneal T cells suggested that subpopulations of regulatory CD4+ Foxp3+ and CD8+ Foxp3+ T cells were involved in modulating the immune responses in the chronic stage of AE, which are Th2 polarized responses (Mejri *et al.*, 2011b).

A primary infection with oncospheres of *E. granulosus* in mice (Zhang *et al.*, 2001) generated a low level antibody response during the first 8 weeks (Zhang *et al.*, 2003b), possibly indicating host immunosuppression. After 9 weeks of the primary infection, antibodies against hydatid cyst fluid and oncosphere antigens were significantly increased, suggesting that antibody production during the course of the infection may be regulated, perhaps through periodic release of antigen from cysts and/or general down regulation of B-cells through T-helper cell activity.

AgB is the most evaluated echinococcal antigen for its role in modulation of immune responses. AgB significantly inhibits polymorphonuclear cell recruitment (Rigano *et al.*, 2001; Shepherd *et al.*, 1991), modulates dendritic cell differentiation and polarizes immature DC maturation towards a Th2 cell response (Rigano *et al.*, 2007). After establishment in the host, the hydatid cyst produces a large amount of AgB (Zhang *et al.*, 2003b), which can alter the Th1/Th2 ratio from a predominant Th1 response in the early stage of infection to a Th2 response (Rigano *et al.*, 2001), indicating that AgB is a modulator of the T cell response benefiting parasite survival. A number of studies have shown that AgB is encoded by a gene family and the antigen exhibits a high degree of genetic polymorphism (Haag *et al.*, 2006; Rosenzvit *et al.*, 2006; Kamenetzky *et al.*, 2005), suggesting that the *Echinococcus* organisms have evolved antigenic variation-type mechanisms for escaping the host immune response.

4. Serological diagnosis of human echinococcosis

Typical asymptomatic features in the early stages of infection and for a long period after establishment makes early diagnosis of echinococcosis in humans difficult. Although the definitive diagnosis for most human cases of CE is by physical imaging methods, such as X-ray, ultrasonography, computed axial tomography (CT scanning) and magnetic resonance imaging, these procedures are often not readily available in isolated communities and usually they provide effective diagnosis mainly of the late development stages of clinical infection. Early diagnosis of CE and AE by serology may, therefore, provide opportunities for early treatment and more effective chemotherapy. Another practical application of serology in human echinococcosis is the follow-up of the treatment. Although hydatid disease is an asymptomatic infection, the host does produce detectable humoral and cellular responses against the infection. Measurement of these responses is a prerequisite for developing effective serodiagnostic tools.

4.1 Methodology in detecting antibodies

Almost all serological tests have been developed for immunodiagnosis of human CE cases. These include indirect haemagglutination (IHA), latex agglutination (LA), complement fixation test (CFT), immunoelectrophoresis (IEP) tests and enzyme-linked immunosorbent assay (ELISA) (Rickard *et al.*, 1984; Rickard, 1984). In contrast, the CFT and LA tests are more likely to give non-specific or false positive reactions (Rickard, 1984) as is the IHA test when serum titres are lower than 1:512 (Varela-Diaz *et al.*, 1975c; Varela-Diaz *et al.*, 1975b; Varela-Diaz *et al.*, 1975a; Craig and Nelson, 1984).

There are considerable differences between the various tests both in specificity and sensitivity. As the sensitivity of a test increases, so generally does the demand for improved antigens in order that sufficient specificity can be achieved to take advantage of the greater sensitivity. An optimum test should be specific with high sensitivity. Insensitive and non-specific tests including the Cassoni intradermal test, CFT, IHA and LA test have been replaced by ELISA, IEP, indirect immunofluorescence antibody test (IFAT), and immunoblotting (IB) in routine laboratory application (Lightowlers and Gottstein, 1995; Nasrieh and Abdel-Hafez, 2004)). ELISA achieved sensitivity rates of 88 to 98% using cyst fluid preparations (Rickard *et al.*, 1984; Speiser, 1980).

Recently developed dipstick assays (van Doorn *et al.*, 2007) are considered to be valuable methods for CE serodiagnosis. A dipstick assay has been developed that exhibited 100% sensitivity and 91.4% specificity with 26 CE sera and 35 other parasite infection sera using camel hydatid cyst fluid as antigen (Al-Sherbiny *et al.*, 2004). Since the dipstick assay is extremely easy to perform with a visually interpreted result within 15 min, in addition to being both sensitive and specific, the test could be an acceptable alternative for use in clinical laboratories lacking specialized equipment and the technological expertise needed for IB or ELISA.

One study (Ortona *et al.*, 2000) highlights the need to standardize techniques and antigenic preparations and to improve the performance of immunodiagnosis by characterizing new antigens and detecting distinct immunoglobulin classes. The diagnostic sensitivity and specificity of IEP, ELISA and IB, in detecting IgG antibodies in patient sera to native and recombinant AgB and a hydatid fluid fraction (HFF) were compared. Sera tested were from patients who had CE grouped according to their type of cysts, from patients with other parasitic diseases, lung or liver carcinomas or serous cysts, and from healthy controls. HFF-IB gave the highest sensitivity (80%) followed by ELISA (72%) and IEP (31%). The diagnostic sensitivity significantly decreased as cysts matured (from type I-II to type VII, classified by ultrasound). Recombinant and native AgB-IB yielded similar sensitivity (74%) but a large number of clinically or surgically confirmed CE patients (20%) were negative. In these patient sera, IB to assess the usefulness of another recombinant *E. granulosus* molecule (elongation factor-1 beta/delta) in detecting IgE antibodies, yielded 33% of positivity.

The results of this and other studies suggest that hydatid serology may be improved by combining several defined antigens (including synthetic peptides), and the design of new *E. granulosus*-specific peptides that react with otherwise false-negative sera.

4.2 Immunodiagnosis of cystic echinococcosis in humans

The immunodiagnosis of echinococcosis has been comprehensively reviewed (Zhang *et al.*, 2003a). Over the past decade, diagnosis of CE has improved due to the use of new or more optimal methods for purification of *Echinococcus* antigens from somatic materials, by the application of molecular tools for parasite identification and the synthesis of recombinant diagnostic antigens and immunogenic peptides. These approaches have not only improved the sensitivity and specificity of tests for diagnosis of CE but they have also allowed more reliable characterization of the biological status of parasite materials (Zhang and McManus, 2006; Siles-Lucas and Gottstein, 2001).

The long history of CE serodiagnosis has mainly involved the identification and characterization of specific *E. granulosus* antigens. The lipoproteins antigen B (AgB) and antigen 5 (Ag5), the major components of HCF, have been the two molecules that have received wide attention in regards to diagnosis. Both antigens have been well characterized in terms of their molecular features and diagnostic potential (Zhang *et al.*, 2003a). Although AgB and Ag5 have proved to be diagnostically valuable, there are difficulties related to their lack of sensitivity and specificity and problems with the standardization of their use. Cross-reactivity with antigens from other parasites, notably other taeniid cestodes, is a major problem. IgE cross-reaction with other parasites (Wattal *et al.*, 1988; Force *et al.*, 1992) is common.

Data in the literature for sensitivity and cross-reactivity of serum anti-*Echinococcus* IgE differ significantly; most studies report high specificity (99–100%) (Marinova *et al.*, 2011; Chamekh *et al.*, 1992; Khabiri *et al.*, 2006; Afferni *et al.*, 1984; Sjolander *et al.*, 1989; Zarzosa *et al.*, 1999)

A recent study using a large panel of sera showed that crude or purified antigens from parasite or hydatid cyst fluid generated a reasonable high specificity (Feng *et al.*, 2010). By using 857 sera from confirmed CE patients and 42 sera from AE patients and 697 sera with different infection and medical conditions showed an overall of 93.4% of specificity with relative low sensitivity 57.4-68.4% (Table 1) (Feng *et al.*, 2010).

Antigen	Test	Number of subjects tested CE	Healthy	Other diseases	Sensitivity (%)	Specificity (%)	Reference
HBLF	LA	119	37	54	86	87.9	(Barbieri *et al.*, 1993)
HFF	IHA	204	90	53	54	100	(Ortona *et al.*, 2000)
HFF	IgE IB	204	90	53	80	96	(Ortona *et al.*, 2000)
HFF	IEP	204	90	53	31	100	(Ortona *et al.*, 2000)
HCF	IgG ELISA	71	45	62	64	80	(Verastegui *et al.*, 1992)
FBHCF	IgG ELISA	119	37	54	83	86.8	(Barbieri *et al.*, 1993)
sWHF	IgG ELISA	111/Li	0	0	89	nd	(Babba *et al.*, 1994)
sWHF	IgG ELISA	122/Lu	0	0	78	nd	(Babba *et al.*, 1994)
FBHCF	IgG ELISA	90	28	88	84	60	(Barbieri *et al.*, 1998)
HCF	IgG ELISA	87	200	339	94	82.3	(Poretti *et al.*, 1999)
HCF	IgG ELISA	42	15	41	81	95	(Irabuena *et al.*, 2000)
HFF	IgG ELISA	204	90	53	72	97	(Ortona *et al.*, 2000)
ppHCF	IgG ELISA	70	30	73	89	40.8	(Jiang *et al.*, 2001)
HCF	IgG ELISA	129	203	65	78	97	(Virginio *et al.*, 2003)
HCF	IgG ELISA	59	15	55	79	73	(Lorenzo *et al.*, 2005)
HCF	IgG ELISA	26	10	45	96	100	(Al-Sherbiny *et al.*, 2004)
HCF	IgG Dip	26	10	45	100	91	(Al-Sherbiny *et al.*, 2004)
HCF	IgG WB	71	45	62	65	91	(Verastegui *et al.*, 1992)
HCF AgB	IgG Dot-IB	875	5	739	68.4	93.4	(Feng *et al.*, 2010)
HCF AgB	IgG ELISA	857	5	739	57.4	93.4	(Feng *et al.*, 2010)
HCF AgB	IgE WB	324	70	500	86.4	92	(Li *et al.*, 2003b)
HCF	IgG WB	26	10	45	100	91	(Al-Sherbiny *et al.*, 2004)
HCF	IgE ImCAP	155	110	58	73.6	99.1	(Marinova *et al.*, 2011)
HCF	IgG ELISA	155	110	58	90.3	90.9	(Marinova *et al.*, 2011)
HCF	IgG WB	155	110	58	90.1	94.5	(Marinova *et al.*, 2011)

Table 1. Features of assays for immunodiagnosis of cystic echinococcosis based on hydatid cyst fluid antigens and native proteins from *E. granulosus* Abbreviations: HFF - hydatid fluid fraction, rich in Ag5 and AgB; HBLF - heparin-binding lipoprotein fraction; ppHCF - partially purified HCF; FBHCF - fertile bovine hydatid cyst fluid; Li - liver; Lu - lung; sWHF - sheep whole hydatid cyst fluid; IHA - indirect haemagglutination assay; LA - Latex agglutination assay; IEP - immunoelectrophoresis; ELISA - enzyme - linked immunosorbent assay; WB - Western blotting; Dip, dipstick; ImCAP, immunoCAP system.

4.2.1 *E. granulosus* antigen B

E. granulosus antigen B (AgB), a polymeric lipoprotein with a molecular weight of 120 kDa, is a highly immunogenic molecule, a characteristic that underpins its value in serodiagnosis (Table 2). AgB can be measured in patient blood as circulating antigen (Kanwar *et al.*, 1994; Kanwar and Kanwar, 1994; Liu *et al.*, 1993). It has a molecular size of circa 8 kDa on sodium dodecyl sulfate polyacrylamide gel electrophoresis (SDS-PAGE) (Lightowlers *et al.*, 1989; Shepherd and McManus, 1987) under reduced conditions. The function of AgB in the parasite's biology is not completely elucidated, but several studies have shown that the molecule may be involved in the modulation of the host immune response; for instance, as a protease inhibitor that inhibits neutrophil chemotaxis (Shepherd *et al.*, 1991; Virginio *et al.*, 2007), promoting a non-protective Th2 response by interfering with monocyte differentiation, and by modulating DC maturation (Kanan and Chain, 2006; Rigano *et al.*, 2007). One study has suggested that AgB could be involved in the processes of lipid uptake or detoxification (Chemale *et al.*, 2005).

AgB	Test	Number of subjects tested			Sensitivity (%)	Specificity (%)	Reference
		CE	Healthy	Other diseases			
Gel-EF	IgG ELISA	204	90	53	74	100	(Ortona *et al.*, 2000)
pp	IgG ELISA	90	28	86	77	85	(Gonzalez-Sapienza *et al.*, 2000)
pp	IgG ELISA	191	50	133	79	98	(Shambesh *et al.*, 1997)
pp	IgG ELISA	81	-	98	89	86	(Wen and Craig, 1994)
AEC	IgG ELISA	31	29	87	77	82	(Rott *et al.*, 2000)
mAb-AP	IgG ELISA	90	28	88	77	86	(Barbieri *et al.*, 1998)
pp	IgG1 ELISA	81	-	98	58	92	(Wen and Craig, 1994)
pp	IgG1 ELISA	191	50	133	57	100	(Shambesh *et al.*, 1997)
pp	IgG2 ELISA	81	-	98	53	94	(Wen and Craig, 1994)
pp	IgG3 ELISA	81	-	98	46	95	(Wen and Craig, 1994)
pp	IgG4 ELISA	210	47	79	63	81	(McVie *et al.*, 1997)
pp	IgG4 ELISA	191	50	133	38	99	(Shambesh *et al.*, 1997)
pp	IgG4 ELISA	81	-	98	73	91	(Wen and Craig, 1994)
pp	IgG4 ELISA	210	47	79	63	81	(McVie *et al.*, 1997)
AgB	IgG ELISA	129	203	65	60	93	(Virginio *et al.*, 2003)
AgB	IgG ELISA	36	36	-	91.7	97.2	(Kalantari *et al.*, 2010)
AgB	IgG ELISA	59	15	55	80	77	(Lorenzo *et al.*, 2005)
AgB	IgG ELISA	40	70	40	92	97	(Sadjjadi *et al.*, 2007)
pp	IgG dELISA	210	47	79	93	65	(McVie *et al.*, 1997)
18kDa	IgG WB	69	82	63	10	77	(Jiang *et al.*, 2001)
8 kDa	IgG WB	35	200	339	71	97	(Poretti *et al.*, 1999)
8 kDa	IgG WB	52p	200	339	60	97	(Poretti *et al.*, 1999)
8-34kDa	IgG WB	173	29	66(AE)	85	65	(Ito *et al.*, 1999)
8-34kDa	IgG WB	35	200	339	91	94	(Poretti *et al.*, 1999)
8-34kDa	IgG WB	52p	200	339	81	94	(Poretti *et al.*, 1999)
Gel-EF	IgG WB	204	90	53	66	100	(Ortona *et al.*, 2000)
pp	IgG WB	158	29	152	92	69	(Ito *et al.*, 1999)
pp	IgG WB	173	29	115	92	100	(Ito *et al.*, 1999)
8kDa	IgG WB	44	-	43	47.7	51.2	(de la Rue *et al.*, 2010)
16kDa	IgG WB	44	-	43	45.5	67.4	(de la Rue *et al.*, 2010)
24kDa	IgG WB	44	-	43	68.2	62.8	(de la Rue *et al.*, 2010)

Table 2. Features of assays for immunodiagnosis of cystic echinococcosis using native antigen B Abbreviations: Gel-EF - eluted fractions from SDS-PAGE; pp - partial purification; AEC - anion exchange chromatography; mAb - AP - affinity purification by monoclonal antibody; 52p - days post-surgery; AE - alveolar echinococcosis; ELISA - enzyme - linked immunosorbent assay; dELISA - dot - ELISA; WB - Western blot.

AgB is a gene family containing at least 10 genes in 5 subfamilies (Shepherd *et al.*, 1991; Fernandez *et al.*, 1996; Chemale *et al.*, 2001; Arend *et al.*, 2004; Mamuti *et al.*, 2007; Zhang *et al.*, 2010), which are differentially expressed in different stages of *E. granulosus* (Mamuti *et al.*, 2007; Zhang *et al.*, 2010). Several AgB cDNAs, such as rAgB8/1 and rAgB8/2, have been cloned, expressed as recombinant proteins and used for diagnosis. AgB8/2 provided the highest diagnostic sensitivity (84-93.1%) and specificity (98-99.5%) (Rott *et al.*, 2000; Virginio *et al.*, 2003). Furthermore, the IgG4 response against AgB appears to be the subclass of choice for serological testing (Siracusano *et al.*, 2004).

The sensitivity and specificity of native *E. granulosus* cyst fluid antigens and native and recombinant AgB are shown in Tables 1-3. These studies used small panel of sera and

Antigen	**Assay method**	**Number of subjects tested**			**Sensitivity (%)**	**Specificity (%)**	**Reference**
		CE	**Healthy**	**Other diseases**			
rAgB.MBP	IgG4 ELISA	210	47	79	65	91	(McVie *et al.*, 1997)
EG55-GST	IgG ELISA	64	39	105	89	72	(Helbig *et al.*, 1993)
rAgB8/1	IgG ELISA	31	29	87	55	80	(Rott *et al.*, 2000)
rAgB8/2	IgG ELISA	31	29	87	84	98	(Rott *et al.*, 2000)
rEgPS-3-GST	IgG ELISA	119	44	123	74	87	(Leggatt and McManus, 1994)
P176	IgG ELISA	90	28	86	80	93	(Gonzalez-Sapienza *et al.*, 2000)
P175	IgG ELISA	90	28	86	49	94	(Gonzalez-Sapienza *et al.*, 2000)
P177	IgG ELISA	90	28	86	38	92	(Gonzalez-Sapienza *et al.*, 2000)
P65	IgG ELISA	90	28	86	44	96	(Gonzalez-Sapienza *et al.*, 2000)
pGu4	IgG ELISA	90	28	86	18	98	(Gonzalez-Sapienza *et al.*, 2000)
pGU4	IgG ELISA	31	29	87	26	-	(Rott *et al.*, 2000)
p65#	IgG ELISA	90	28	88	34-48	80-97	(Barbieri *et al.*, 1998)
pGU4#	IgG ELISA	90	28	88	12-18	96-100	(Barbieri *et al.*, 1998)
rAgB.MBP	IgG dELISA	210	47	79	74	88	(McVie *et al.*, 1997)
p65	IgG dELISA	25	9	8	64	100	(Leggatt and McManus, 1994)
rAgB-GST	IgG WB	204	90	53	72	100	(Ortona *et al.*, 2000)
P176	IgG ELISA	59	15	55	63	82	
rAgB1		59	15	55	68	88	(Lorenzo *et al.*, 2005)
rAgB1	IgG ELISA	102	95	68	88.2	80.9	(Hernandez-Gonzalez *et al.*, 2008)
rAgB2	IgG ELISA	102	95	68	91.2	93	(Hernandez-Gonzalez *et al.*, 2008)
rAgB-GST	IgG IB	120	24	97	79.2	81	(Lv *et al.*, 2009)
rAgB	IgG ELISA	246		173	77.6		(Li *et al.*, 2010)

Table 3. Features of assays for immunodiagnosis of cystic echinococcosis based on using recombinant antigen B and antigen B peptides Abbreviations: ELISA - enzyme-linked immunosorbent assay; dELISA - dot enzyme - linked immunosorbent assay; ELISAs - sandwich ELISA; rEgPS - recombinant protoscolex protein; GST- glutathione *S*-transferase; rAgB - recombinant antigen B; MBP - maltose binding protein; # - coated with different buffer; WB-Western blot

showed generally both high sensitivity and specificity (Tawfeek *et al.*, 2011; Kalantari *et al.*, 2010; Abdi *et al.*, 2010; Lv *et al.*, 2009; Sadjjadi *et al.*, 2007; Virginio *et al.*, 2003). Cross-reactions, mainly with sera from AE patients, have been reported to be up to 47.7% (de la Rue *et al.*, 2010).

In addition, a number of AgB peptides have been synthesized and used in ELISA for diagnostic purposes (Table 3). Peptide antigens have been considered as a way to enhance specificity and efforts have been made to define discrete epitopes of AgB and other molecules that could be mimicked by synthetic peptides. However, a double-blind, randomized multicenter comparison of the diagnostic performance of six major antigens (namely, HCF, native AgB, two recombinant AgB subunits, an AgB-derived synthetic peptide, and recombinant cytosolic malate dehydrogenase) against the same serum collection showed the AgB-derived synthetic peptide provided relatively poor specificity, with instead, one of the recombinant AgB subunits (AgB8/1) being recommended as the standard antigen for laboratory analysis (Lorenzo *et al.*, 2005).

4.2.2 *E. granulosus* antigen 5

E. granulosus antigen 5 (Ag5) is a very high molecular weight (approximately 400 kDa) lipoprotein complex composed of 57- and 67-kDa components that, under reducing conditions, dissociate into 38- and 22- to 24-kDa subunits in SDS-PAGE. Historically, one of the most used immunodiagnostic procedures for CE was the demonstration of serum antibodies precipitating antigen 5 (arc 5) by immunoelectrophoresis or similar techniques. Table 4 shows the performance of antigen 5 for serological diagnosis of human CE. Loss of sugar determinants on antigen 5 can reduce the antigenicity of the native protein (Lorenzo et al., 2005a). The potential value of specific antibodies of different IgG subclasses and IgE in serological diagnosis of CE using an ELISA based on Ag5 has been evaluated (Khabiri et al., 2006). The presence of IgG1 was demonstrated in all sera from 58 patients with CE. The most discriminatory and specific antibodies found in this study were IgG4 and IgE. Only one false-positive reaction was observed with IgG4 and no IgE cross-reactivity occurred with 40 sera from healthy controls. In 36 sera from patients with parasitic diseases other than CE, two false-positive reactions with IgG4 were observed but none occurred with IgE. In immunoblotting, it was shown that the IgG1 subclass was responsible for cross-reactivity of human antibodies that reacted with the 38kDa subunit of Ag5. IgG4 and IgE antibodies could not recognize the 38kDa subunit and under non-reducing conditions reacted with the 57kDa subunit without any cross-reactivity with other parasites. These results demonstrated that IgG4 and IgE are the most important antibodies for serological diagnosis of CE in an Ag5-based immunoassay system. Like AgB, Ag5 has been cloned, expressed and tested for diagnostic performance but the recombinant protein showed low sensitivity (Table 4).

4.2.3 Other recombinant proteins and approaches for immunodiagnosis

Table 4 lists the diagnostic performance of some other recombinant *E. granulosus* proteins cloned recently. Li et al. (2003b) cloned a fragment designated as EpC1 and tested 896 human serum samples including 324 sera samples from patients with CE, 172 from patients with neurocysticercosis, 89 from patients with AE, and 241 from patients with other infections or clinical presentations, as well as 70 from confirmed-negative control subjects.

Antigen	Test	Number of objects tested			Sensitivity (%)	Specificity (%)	Reference
		CE	Heathy	Other disease			
Arc5	IEP	35	200	289	63	97.2	(Poretti et al., 1999)
Arc5	IEP	52p*	200	289	58	97.2	(Poretti et al., 1999)
mAb-AP	IgG ELISA	90	28	88	50	92	(Barbieri et al., 1998)
mAb-AP	IgG ELISA	39	29	51	54	89	(Gonzalez et al., 2000)
P89-122#	IgG ELISA	90	28	88	14-21	77-100	(Barbieri et al., 1998)
rP-29	IgG ELISA	39	29	51	61	80	(Gonzalez et al., 2000)
P89-122#	IgG ELISA	39	29	51	44	100	(Gonzalez et al., 2000)
pAg 5	IgG ELISA	111(Li)	nd	nd	89	nd	(Babba et al., 1994)
pAg 5	IgG ELISA	122(Lu)	nd	nd	78	nd	(Babba et al., 1994)
nAg5	IgG ELISA	58	40	36	100	70.2	(Khabiri et al., 2006)
nAg5	IgG1 ELISA	58	40	36	100	70.2	(Khabiri et al., 2006)
nAg5	IgG4 ELISA	58	40	36	75.8	93	(Khabiri et al., 2006)
nAg5	IgE ELISA	58	40	36	70	100	(Khabiri et al., 2006)
rAg5	IgG ELISA	34	18	36	65	89	(Lorenzo et al., 2005b)
rAg5-38	IgG ELISA	34	18	36	21	97	(Lorenzo et al., 2005b)
EpC1	IgG WB	324	70	500	88.7	95.6	(Li et al., 2003b)
rEgcMDH	IgG ELISA	59	15	55	45	83	(Lorenzo et al., 2005a)
HSP20	IgG1/4 WB	95	37	-	64	-	(Vacirca et al., 2011)
Eg19	IgG WB	97	37	58	10	100	(Delunardo et al., 2010)
E14t	IgG ELISA	102	95	68	35.3	91.7	(Hernandez-Gonzalez et al., 2008)
C317	IgG ELISA	102	95	68	58.8	80.9	(Hernandez-Gonzalez et al., 2008)
P5	IgG WB	60	-	-	97	-	(Zhang et al., 2007)

* post-treatment. Abbreviations: Li - liver; Lu - lung; mAb-AP - affinity purified using monoclonal antibody; # - coated with different buffer; pAg5 - purified antigen 5; nd - not determined.

Table 4. Features of assays for immunodiagnosis of cystic echinococcosis based on using native, recombinant and synthetic peptides of antigen 5 and other proteins

The fusion protein yielded an overall sensitivity of 92.2% and an overall specificity of 95.6%. The combined levels of sensitivity and specificity achieved with the rEpC1-GST fusion protein for diagnosis of CE were exceptional, taking into account the large panel of serum samples that were tested (Li et al., 2003b). The cDNA sequence coding for EpC1 has high amino acid sequence identity to a paralogue from *Taenia solium*, the cause of neurocysticercosis (NCC). To determine diagnostic antibody-binding regions on EpC1 recognized specifically by CE sera, 10 truncated regions (P1-10) of the immunogenic protein were expressed in Escherichia coli and subjected to immunoblotting (Zhang et al., 2007). One peptide, designated peptide 5 (P5, fused with glutathione-S-transferase (GST)) was positively recognized by sera from mice experimentally infected with oncospheres of *E. granulosus* and sera from surgically confirmed CE patients. Sera from NCC patients did not react with any of the peptides used. There are four amino acid substitutions in P5 compared with the T. solium sequence and these may form part of the epitope inducing CE-specific antibody. Ninety-seven per cent (58 of 60) of sera from confirmed CE patients recognized P5-GST.

By using ELISA, a cytosolic isoform of malate dehydrogenase (EgcMDH), an EF-hand calcium-binding protein (EgCaBP2), and a full-length (EgAFFPf) and a truncated form

(EgAFFPt, aa 261 370) of actin yielded sensitivities between 58.6% and 89.7%, and three of them were considered of complementary value (Virginio et al., 2003).

A purified alkaline phosphatase (EgAP) extracted from *E. granulosus* hydatid cyst membranes has shown exceptional diagnostic characteristics with 100% specificity without any decrease in sensitivity (100%) with significant potential for use in routine diagnosis and follow-up of CE patients (Mahmoud and Abou Gamra, 2004). This mirrors the diagnostic value previously shown for purified alkaline phosphatase (pAP) from *E. multilocularis* metacestodes (Zhang et al., 2003a).

Purified recombinant thioredoxin peroxidase from *E. granulosus* (TPxEg) was used to screen sera from heavily infected mice and patients with confirmed hydatid infection (Li *et al.*, 2004). Only a portion of the sera reacted positively with the EgTPx-GST fusion protein in Western blots (69.3% specificity and 39% sensitivity with human sera), suggesting that EgTPx may form antibody-antigen complexes or that responses to the EgTPx antigen may be immunologically regulated.

IB revealed anti-HSP20 antibodies in a higher percentage of sera from patients with active disease than in sera from patients with inactive disease (Vacirca *et al.*, 2011). A comparison of the ImmunoCAP system for testing serum IgE compared with IgG-ELISA and IgG-Western blotting revealed the former test had a higher specificity and lower cross-reactivity with a sensitivity of 73.6% (Marinova *et al.*, 2011).

4.3 Immunodiagnosis of alveolar echinococcosis in humans

A number of advances in the serodiagnosis of AE have occurred in the past 10 years or so. These include identification of novel antigens, such as Em2 and Em18. Em2 was purified originally from *E. multilocularis* metacestode tissue extracts by affinity chromatography (Gottstein, 1985). Using AE sera to screen a cDNA library, a clone termed II/3 was cloned and showed very high performance for diagnosis (Vogel *et al.*, 1988). A commerical kit based on Em2 and recombinant truncted protein II/3 so called Em2 ^{Plus} ELISA has shown high performance of AE diagnosis (Gottstein *et al.*, 1993).

Em18, an 18-kD antigen from *E. multilocularis,* is highly specific for detection of AE (Ito *et al.*, 2003a; Xiao *et al.*, 2003). An ELISA system using the recombinant Em18 antigen (RecEm18) could differentially distinguish AE from CE (Ito *et al.*, 2003a) and may be used for monitering surgical and/or chemotherapeutic treatment and the follow up of AE patients after treatment (Fujimoto *et al.*, 2005). In order to compare the sequential responses of IgG subclasses to Em18 in sera from patients with AE, a total of 225 sera from 36 patients at different clinical stages according to the WHO-PNM staging system (Pawlowski *et al.*, 2001) were tested. The levels of serum IgG and IgG4 against Em18 correlated with the PNM stages compared with sera from patients receiving no treatment (Tappe *et al.*, 2010).

Antibody-screening was performed by (Reiter-Owona *et al.*, 2009) using ELISA, IHA and IFAT, and confirmatory testing was done using the commercialized *E. multilocularis*-specific Em2plus-ELISA versus an in-house *E. multilocularis*-specific Em10-ELISA. The study showed that the Em2plus-ELISA reacted with 23.5% CE-positive sera, whereas the Em10-ELISA did not exhibit any cross-reactivity. In sera from patients with AE, confirmation by both ELISAs was achieved in 57.6% of cases, mostly in patients with an advanced stage of the disease and high antibody titers in the screening assays. False-negative reactions with both ELISAs occurred in 30.3% cases, mostly in patients who had low antibody levels in the screening tests. The Em2plus-ELISA exhibited fewer false-negative reactions than the Em10-ELISA. WB confirmed the positive results of both assays and was the assay with the highest reliability with different stages of CE and AE, followed by the Em2plus-ELISA for AE. High antibody titres in the screening assays favour the detection of species-specific antibodies to either CE or AE (Reiter-Owona *et al.*, 2009). The features of assays currently available for immunodiagnosis of alveolar echinococcosis using different antigens are presented in Table 5.

Antigen	TEST	Number of subjects tested			Sensitivity (%)	Specificity (%)	Reference
		AE	Healthy	Other disease			
Em2^{plus}	IgG ELISA	140	500	400	97.1	90.2	(Gottstein *et al.*, 1993)
Em2	IgG ELISA	140	500	400	89.3	98.0	(Gottstein *et al.*, 1993)
Em2^{plus}	IgG ELISA	47	-	-	81	-	(Bart *et al.*, 2007)
Em2	IgG ELISA	62	-	97	90	65	(Muller *et al.*, 2007)
rEm10	IgG ELISA	74	39	95	93.2	96.5	(Helbig *et al.*, 1993)
II/3-10	IgG ELISA	140	500	400	86.4	96.8	(Gottstein *et al.*, 1993)
CH-10	IgG ELISA	140	500	400	96	39-97	(Gottstein *et al.*, 1993)
N3C	IgG ELISA	140	500	400	96	18-94	(Gottstein *et al.*, 1993)
pAP	IgG ELISA	37	37	95	100	100	(Ravinder *et al.*, 1997)
Em70	IgG ELISA	39	32	115	100	99	(Korkmaz *et al.*, 2004)
Em90	IgG ELISA	39	32	115	100	99	(Korkmaz *et al.*, 2004)
II/3-10	IgG ELISA	62	-	97	79	92	(Muller *et al.*, 2007)
Em18	IgG ELISA	44	30	99	91	89.1	(Jiang *et al.*, 2001)
rEm13	IgG ELISA	28	-	72	82.1	100	(Frosch *et al.*, 1993)
rEm18	IgG IB	66	29	259	97	96.9	(Ito *et al.*, 1999)
rEm18	IgG IB	33	82	99	91	92.3	(Jiang *et al.*, 2001)
rEm18	ELISA	19	0	189	100	99	(Xiao *et al.*, 2003)
EmII	Dot-IB	42	-	-	91.1	-	(Feng *et al.*, 2010)

Table 5. Features of assays for immunodiagnosis of alveolar echinococcosis using different antigens

Although AE serological diagnosis has made great strides to practical application, a recent expert consensus for alveolar echinococcosis diagnosis (Brunetti *et al.*, 2010) stated that the most patients with AE are diagnosed at a later stage, which significantly impacts on quality of treatment. There is an urgent need for the early diagnosis. The application of new techniques is a way to address these issues; for example, recent microarray analysis identified 5 genes (Gapdh, Est1, Rlp3, Mdh-1, Rpl37) exhibiting a high level of congruency, and these may provide new diagnostic targets to predict disease status and progression (Gottstein *et al.*, 2010).

4.4 Circulating antigen detection

Antibody detection is likely to indicate exposure to an *Echinococcus* infection, but it may not necessarily point to the presence of an established, viable infection, or the disease. Serum antibodies may persist for a prolonged period, reaching up to 10 years after hydatid cyst removal (Li *et al.*, 2004). In addition, the degree of antibody response may be related to the location and condition of a mature hydatid cyst. For instance, hydatid cysts in human lung, spleen, or kidney tend to be associated with lower serum antibody levels (Zhang and McManus, 2006). Furthermore, in *Echinococcus*-endemic villages, up to 26% or more of the general population may have antibodies to HCF antigens, but with only about 2% of the villagers having hydatid cysts (Craig *et al.*, 1986; Chai *et al.*, 1989; Gavidia *et al.*, 2008), indicating that the antibody levels may not necessarily reflect the true prevalence of CE.

Antigen detection assays depend principally on the binding of specific polyclonal or monoclonal antibodies to parasite antigen present in serum or urine. A number of different assays have been developed to detect echinococcal antigens. The standard double antibody sandwich ELISA is a common method for measuring the presence and/or concentration of circulating parasite antigens. In the test, antibody raised to the targeted protein is coated onto a microtiter plate to capture antigen (Fig 3). The same antibody, that is enzyme labeled, is commonly used in the tertiary layer of the assay. This type of antigen capture therefore relies on the presence of multiple binding sites on the target antigens(s). Efforts to detect CAg in CE patients have been reviewed extensively by Craig (Craig *et al.*, 1986).

CAg in serum is normally in the form of a circulating immune complex (CIC) with some in free form. Therefore, the serum needs to be treated with acid buffer or polyethylene glycol (PEG) to release and concentrate the circulating antigens. Acidic treatment (0.2 M glycine/HCl) of CE patient serum is quite straightforward to dissociate CIC (Craig *et al.*, 1986). In a comparison of acid-treatment and PEG precipitation methods, all the sera of 30 confirmed positive cases of CE had detectable levels of antigen in the acid-treated sera (Craig, 1993). However, 23 (77%) and 26 (87%) sera of 30 confirmed cases had free antigen as well as CIC of an 8 kDa antigen in the untreated and in the PEG precipitated sera, respectively. None of the sera from other patients with parasitic infections or viral hepatitis had any detectable levels of 8 kDa antigen in the untreated, acid-treated or PEG-precipitated serum samples. These investigations, therefore, suggested that the demonstration of circulating antigen employing monospecific antibodies to affinity purified 8 kDa antigen in acid-treated sera is more efficient than the detection of free circulating antigen or CIC in untreated or in PEG-precipitated sera (Kanwar *et al.*, 1994).

IgM CICs tend to be positively associated with active hydatid disease (Craig *et al.*, 1986; Matossian *et al.*, 1992). Combining measurement of circulating antibody, CICs and CAg resulted in an increase from 77% to 90% compared to measurement of serum antibody alone (Moosa and Abdel-Hafez, 1994). Antigens in soluble CICs from CE patients have been characterized by separating them on SDS-PAGE (Craig *et al.*, 1986) or by ion-exchange fast protein liquid chromatography (FPLC)(Bonifacino *et al.*, 1993). Both studies indicated a candidate antigen detectable in serum with an approximate relative molecular mass of 60-67 KDa, and which is also present in cyst fluid.

Comparison of CAg and IgG antibody using ELISA, together with Western blotting, showed a relatively low sensitivity (43%) for detection of specific serum antigen in CE, compared to 75% for IgG antibodies (Craig, 1997). However, the specificity of this CAg ELISA was 90% when tested against sera from AE patients and 100% against human cysticercosis sera. The limited cross-reactivity may be a way for practical diagnosis of CE in areas where AE and cysticercosis are co-endemic. The advantage of CAg detection is its high sensitivity for detecting CE in 54-57% of patients who are serum antibody negative (Moosa and Abdel-Hafez, 1994; Craig, 1997). CAg detection does appear, therefore, to be potentially useful as a secondary test for some suspected CE cases where antibody titers are low (Craig *et al.*, 1986; Schantz, 1988).

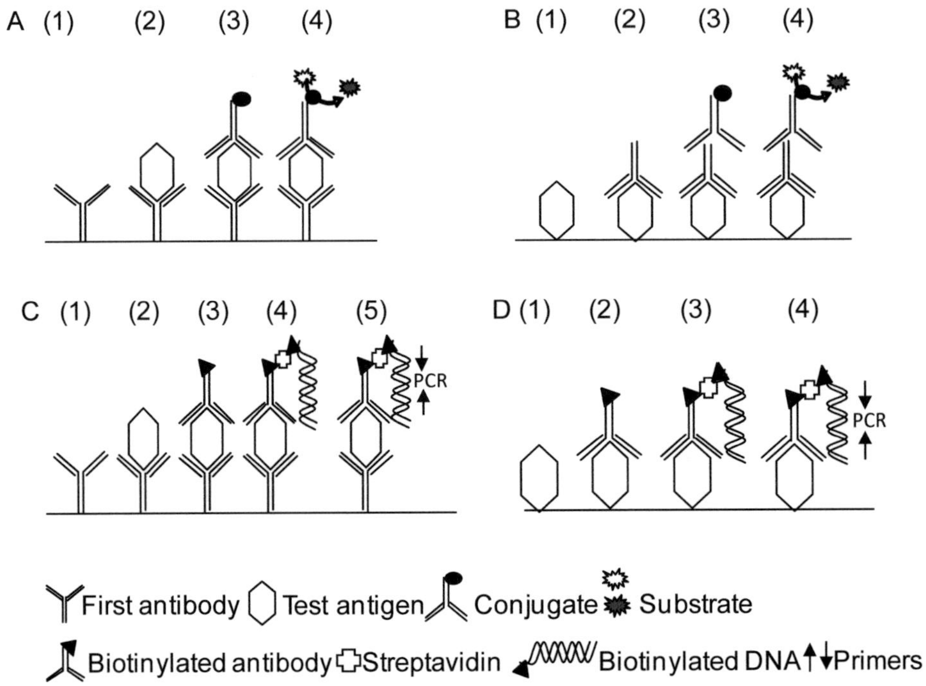

Fig. 3. Schematic of ELISA and immuno-PCR for detecting circulating antigen in serum. A. Sandwich ELISA. (1) Plate is coated with a capture antibody; (2) Serum sample is added, and any antigen present in the serum binds to the capture antibody; (3) Detecting antibody conjugate is added and binds to the antigen; (4) Substrate is added, and is converted by the enzyme to a detectable form. B. Direct ELISA. Plate is coated with diluted serum containing antigen; (2) Detecting antibody is added, and binds to antigen; (3) Enzyme-linked secondary antibody is added, and binds to detecting antibody; (4) Substrate is added, and is converted by the enzyme to a detectable form. C. Capture immuno-PCR. (1) Plate is coated with capture antibody; (2) Serum sample is added; (3) Biotinylated detecting antibody is added and binds to antigen; (4) Streptavidin and biotinylated reporter DNA are added, and the biotinylated antibody and biotinylated reporter DNA are linked by streptavidin; (5) Primers and PCR components are added and PCR or real- time PCR undertaken to quantify antigen. D, Non-capture immuno-PCR. Serum sample is coated on the plate and the remainder of the steps are as for the capture-imuno-PCR (C).

A combination of CAg and antibody detection has been shown to increase the sensitivity from 85% (antibody only) to 89% (antibody+CAg) in ELISA of 115 surgically confirmed hydatid patients, 41 individuals exhibiting other parasitic and unrelated diseases, and 69 healthy subjects(Barbieri *et al.*, 1994).

Urinary hydatid antigen detection by co-agglutination (Co-A) potentially represents a cost-effective and rapid test for diagnosis of CE in a rural or field setting. However, the lower sensitivity of Co-A for detection of antigen in the urine of a patient whose serum was positive for the antigen is possibly due to low levels of antigen in the urine (Ravinder *et al.*, 2000).

Although there has been no application to date for echinococcal diagnosis, a technique for antigen detection, called immuno-polymerase chain reaction (immuno-PCR) (Fig 3 C and D), has been developed (Sano *et al.*, 1992). It combines the molecular recognition of antibodies with the high DNA amplification capability of PCR. The procedure is similar to conventional ELISA but is far more sensitive, and, in principle, could be applied for the detection of single antigen molecules. Instead of an enzyme, a DNA molecule is linked to the detection antibody and serves as a template for PCR (Fig 3). The DNA molecule is amplified and the PCR product is measured by gel electrophoresis. An improvement of this method is to amplify the DNA fragment by real-time PCR, thereby eliminating post-PCR analysis. Furthermore, real-time PCR is extremely accurate and sensitive, which should make it possible to quantitate very low amounts of DNA-coupled detection antibody with high accuracy.

5. Immunodiagnosis of cystic echinococcosis in intermediate host animals

Research towards developing serological tests for the diagnosis of larval cestode infection in animals has been largely unsuccessful. Substantial problems remain, due to the frequent existence of multiple infections with different taeniid species, antigenic cross-reactivity between these related parasites, and the low level of specific antibody response to infection. Problems with poor specificity and sensitivity of traditional serological tests for cysticercosis and hydatidosis have prevented the development of any practical test for ante-mortem diagnosis of infection. An approach to the diagnosis of *Taenia* infection by detecting circulating parasite antigen (Onyango-Abuje *et al.*, 1996; Lightowlers, 1990; Harrison *et al.*, 1989) offers some prospect for the development of a practical diagnostic test for cysticercosis.

In comparison with the extensive investigations in humans, relatively little research has been directed toward the development of immunodiagnostic techniques for *E. granulosus* infection in domesticated animals such as sheep and cattle. Currently, diagnosis of CE in intermediate hosts is based mainly on necropsy procedures. However, up to 37% of animals classified as positive at necropsy may be actually false positives caused by unspecific granulomas, pseudo-tuberculosis, fatty degeneration, abscesses, caseous lymphadenitis, and larval stage of *Taenia hydatigena*, whereas false negative diagnoses may be due to small intra-parenchyma cysts (Larrieu *et al.*, 2001; Gatti *et al.*, 2007).

Accurate serological diagnosis of CE infection in livestock is necessary, but, as indicated above, difficult due to serological cross-reactions with several other species of taeniid cestodes including *Taenia hydatigena* and *T.ovis* (Lightowlers and Gottstein, 1995; Yong *et al.*, 1984). Furthermore, natural intermediate host animals produce very poor antibody responses to infection compared with the relatively high levels of specific antibody seen in human infection (Lightowlers and Gottstein, 1995). In sheep, (Lightowlers *et al.*, 1984) detected low levels of antibodies to AgB in the sera of some animals, whereas, others have reported reasonable high antibody responses to this molecule (Kanwar and Kanwar, 1994; Ibrahem *et al.*, 1996). ELISA techniques using a variety of antigens have been applied to the immunodiagnosis of animal CE (Yong *et al.*, 1984). In experimentally infected sheep, antibodies to hydatid antigens can be detected as early as 4-6 weeks post-infection (Yong *et al.*, 1984). However, as referred to above, serological cross-reactions between *E. granulosus* and other cestodes limit the specific diagnosis of hydatid infection by ELISA using crude parasite antigens (Yong *et al.*, 1984). Affinity purification of crude antigens with antibodies from animals immunized with homologous antigen (Craig and Rickard, 1982), or affinity depletion of cross-reactive antigens with monoclonal antibody (Craig *et al.*, 1980), only partially reduces the cross-reactivity. Polysaccharide antigens from either the secretions produced during *in vitro* cultivation of *E. granulosus* PSC or from mouse hydatid cyst membranes by phenol extraction have been used to test sera from sheep (Ris *et al.*, 1987). Although the antibody responses were significantly higher than those of sheep infected with *T. hydatigena* or *T. ovis*, very high cross-reacting antibody responses in the sera from *T. hydatigena*-infected animals were detected with the antigenic secretions from PSC. Neither antigen was sufficiently sensitive or specific for routine serodiagnostic use (Ris *et al.*, 1987).

To develop an immunological method for the identification of sheep infected with *E. granulosus*, (Kittelberger *et al.*, 2002) used an ELISA with antigen comprising either a purified 8 kDa hydatid cyst fluid protein (8kDaELISA), a recombinant EG95 oncosphere protein (OncELISA) or a crude protoscolex preparation (ProtELISA). Sera used for the assay validations were obtained from 249 sheep infected either naturally or experimentally with *E. granulosus* and from 1012 non-infected sheep. The highest diagnostic sensitivity was obtained using the ProtELISA at 62.7 and 51.4%, depending on the cut-off. Assay sensitivities were lower for the 8kDaELISA and the OncELISA. Diagnostic specificities were high, ranging from 95.8 to 99.5%, depending on the ELISA type and cut-off level chosen. A few sera from 39 sheep infected with *T. hydatigena* and from 19 sheep infected with *T. ovis* were recorded as positive. Western immunoblot analysis revealed that the dominant antigenic components in the crude protoscolex antigen preparation were macromolecules of about 70-150 kDa, most likely representing polysaccharides. This study demonstrated that the ProtELISA was the most effective immunological method of those assessed for detection of infection with *E. granulosus* in sheep. Because of its limited diagnostic sensitivity of about 50-60%, it could be useful for the detection of the presence of infected sheep on a flock basis but cannot be used for reliable identification of individual animals infected with *E. granulosus.*

In a later study, Simsek and Koroglu (2004) investigated the antigenic characteristics of hydatid cyst fluid in sheep by SDS-PAGE to evaluate the sensitivity and specificity of HCF-ELISA and immunoblotting for diagnosis of sheep hydatidosis. One band with a molecular weight of 116 kDa showed 88% sensitivity and 84% specificity in the immunoblot assay. Sensitivity (60%) was less but specificity was higher (94%) with the HCF-ELISA (Simsek and Koroglu, 2004). Ghorbanpoor et al. (2006) were able to detect specific circulating antigens or antibodies in the serum and urine of 13 experimentally infected sheep.

6. DNA techniques

In addition to imaging and serological tests, identification of *Echinococcus* infection via PCR-based assays and DNA sequencing using tissue biopsy from the patients can be of choice for confirming diagnosis of echinococcosis for these unconfirmed and complicated cases. DNA techniques are now available that allow the unambiguosus identification of *Echinococcus* species and *E. granulosus* strains using metacestode material excised from intermediate and human hosts provide a major new approach to the diagnosis of echinococcosis (Yang *et al.*, 2006; McManus, 2006; McManus and Thompson, 2003; Thompson and McManus, 2001). Detection or amplification of *E. multilocularis* nucleic acids in clinical samples has been used in diagnosis of AE infections in patients (Myjak *et al.*, 2003).

7. The challenges and future directions

Almost all available immunodiagnostic techniques, including methods for detecting specific antibodies and circulating parasite antigens in serum or other body fluids, have been applied for diagnosing echinococcosis. However, all the tools developed to date, are generally applicable for laboratory research purposes only. None of the available diagnostic tools, kits or methods are generally accepted by clinical physicians. Nevertheless, such serological tools are potentially important for epidemiological studies, confirmation of infection status and the treatment and the monitoring of control programs and efforts should continue so that new assays for improved, practical diagnosis of echinococcosis are developed.

8. Conclusion

This Chapter provides an update of recent progress in research on the immunology and serological diagnosis of echinococcosis caused by *E. granulosus and E. multilocularis.* Cystic echinococcosus (CE) is characterized by long term growth of larval cysts in humans and other intermediate hosts, whereas, alveolar echincoccosis is defined by its chronic progression in human liver, resulting in high mortality. Although the host-parasite interplay, in most cases of AE and CE, appears to be harmonious and clinically asymptomatic for a long period after infection, the host does produce detectable humoral and cellular responses against the causative parasites. Antibody responses against early *E. granulosus* infection are weak being, usually, undetectable in the early two to three weeks following infection. During the establishment stage, the parasite produces significant quantities of antigens that modulate the immune response including antibody production, which is essential for serodiagnostic measurement.

It is clear that the improvement of immunodiagnostic methods for echinococcosis has greatly contributed to a better understanding of the prevalence and the epidemiology of the infection. Immunodiagnostic tests will also provide a valuable tool in measuring the impact of the disease on human health and on animal production, data that are still missing in most endemic areas. The assays may contribute to the diagnosis of CE and AE and the follow-up of treatment. Ultrasound and X-ray imaging methods are generally inaccessible and/or too expensive for the rural population at risk. Under these conditions, serology may provide the only tool for diagnosis of the infection. Finally, efforts should continue to provide cheap, reliable and standardised serodiagnostic methods more widely available for both AE and CE.

9. Acknowledgements

Echinococcosis research projects by the authors are supported by the National Natural Science Foundation of China (30760185 for WBZ, 30960342 and 81160201 for HW) and China

Special Research Projects for Public Sectors (Agriculture), and the Australian National Health and Medical Research Council.

10. References

Abdi, J., Kazemi, B., Mohebali, M., Bandehpour, M., Rahimi, M. T. &Rokni, M. B. (2010). Gene cloning, expression and serological evaluation of the 12-kDa antigen-B subunit from *Echinococcus granulosus*. *Ann Trop Med Parasitol*, Vol.104, No.5, pp. 399-407, ISSN: 1364-8594

Afferni, C., Pini, C., Misiti-Dorello, P., Bernardini, L., Conchedda, M. &Vicari, G. (1984). Detection of specific IgE antibodies in sera from patients with hydatidosis. *Clin Exp Immunol*, Vol.55, No.3, pp.587-592, ISSN:1356-2249, ISSN: 1474-1741

Al-Sherbiny, M. M., Farrag, A. A., Fayad, M. H., Makled, M. K., Tawfeek, G. M. &Ali, N. M. (2004). Application and assessment of a dipstick assay in the diagnosis of hydatidosis and trichinosis. *Parasitol Res*, Vol. 93, No.2, pp. 87-95, ISSN:0932-0113

Allen, J. E. &Maizels, R. M. (2011). Diversity and dialogue in immunity to helminths. *Nat Rev Immunol*, Vol.11, No.6, pp.375-388, ISSN: 1474-1741

Altintas, N. (2003). Past to present: echinococcosis in Turkey. *Acta Trop*, Vol.85, No.2, pp. 105-112, ISSN: 0001-706X

Arend, A. C., Zaha, A., Ayala, F. J. &Haag, K. L. (2004). The *Echinococcus granulosus* antigen B shows a high degree of genetic variability. *Exp Parasitol*. Vol.108, No.1-2, pp. 76-80, ISSN: 0014-4894

Babba, H., Messedi, A., Masmoudi, S., Zribi, M., Grillot, R., Ambriose-Thomas, P., Beyrouti, I. &Sahnoun, Y. (1994). Diagnosis of human hydatidosis: comparison between imagery and six serologic techniques. *Am J Trop Med Hyg*, Vol.50, No.1, pp. 64-68, ISSN: 0002-9637

Barbieri, M., Fernandez, V., Gonzalez, G., Luaces, V. M. &Nieto, A. (1998). Diagnostic evaluation of a synthetic peptide derived from a novel antigen B subunit as related to other available peptides and native antigens used for serology of cystic hydatidosis. *Parasite Immunol*, Vol.20, No.2, pp. 51-61, ISSN: 1365-3024

Barbieri, M., Severi, M. A., Pirez, M. I., Battistoni, J. &Nieto, A. (1994). Use of specific antibody and circulating antigen serum levels in the hydatid immunodiagnosis of asymptomatic population. *Int J Parasitol*, Vol. 24, No.7, pp. 937-942, ISSN: 0020-7519

Barbieri, M., Sterla, S., Battistoni, J. &Nieto, A. (1993). High performance latex reagent for hydatid serology using an *Echinococcus granulosus* lipoprotein antigen fraction purified from cyst fluid in one step. *Int J Parasitol*, Vol.23, No.5, pp.565-572, ISSN: 0020-7519

Bart, J. M., Piarroux, M., Sako, Y., Grenouillet, F., Bresson-Hadni, S., Piarroux, R. &Ito, A. (2007). Comparison of several commercial serologic kits and Em18 serology for detection of human alveolar echinococcosis. *Diagn Microbiol Infect Dis*, Vol.59, No.1, pp. 93-95, ISSN: 0732-8893

Bauder, B., Auer, H., Schilcher, F., Gabler, C., Romig, T., Bilger, B. &Aspock, H. (1999). Experimental investigations on the B and T cell immune response in primary alveolar echinococcosis. *Parasite Immunol*, Vol.21, No.8, pp. 409-421, ISSN: 1365-3024

Bayraktar, M. R., Mehmet, N. &Durmaz, R. (2005). Th1 and Th2 inducing cytokines in Cystic echinococcosis. *Turkiye Parazitol Derg*, Vol.29, No.3, pp.167-170.

Baz, A., Carol, H., Fernandez, V., Mourglia-Ettlin, G., Nieto, A., Orn, A. &Dematteis, S. (2008). *Echinococcus granulosus*: induction of T-independent antibody response against protoscolex glycoconjugates in early experimental infection. *Exp Parasitol*, Vol.119, No.4, pp. 460-466, ISSN: 0014-4894

Baz, A., Ettlin, G. M. &Dematteis, S. (2006). Complexity and function of cytokine responses in experimental infection by *Echinococcus granulosus*. *Immunobiology*, Vol.211, No.1-2, pp. 3-9, ISSN: 0171-2985

Ben Nouir, N., Nunez, S., Gianinazzi, C., Gorcii, M., Muller, N., Nouri, A., Babba, H. &Gottstein, B. (2008). Assessment of *Echinococcus granulosus* somatic protoscolex antigens for serological follow-up of young patients surgically treated for cystic echinococcosis. *J Clin Microbiol*, Vol.46, No.5, pp. 1631-1640, ISSN: 1098-660X

Bonifacino, R., Craig, P., Carter, S., Malgor, R. &Dixon, J. (1993). Partial characterization of antigens in circulating immune complexes in cystic hydatid patients treated with albendazole. *Trans R Soc Trop Med Hyg*, Vol. 87, No.1, pp. 97-102, ISSN: 0035-9203

Bresson-Hadni, S., Liance, M., Meyer, J. P., Houin, R., Bresson, J. L. &Vuitton, D. A. (1990). Cellular immunity in experimental *Echinococcus multilocularis* infection. II. Sequential and comparative phenotypic study of the periparasitic mononuclear cells in resistant and sensitive mice. *Clin Exp Immunol*, Vol.82, No.2, pp. 378-383, ISSN: 1474-1741

Brunetti, E., Kern, P. &Vuitton, D. A. (2010). Expert consensus for the diagnosis and treatment of cystic and alveolar echinococcosis in humans. *Acta Trop*, Vol.114, No.1, pp. 1-16, ISSN: 0001-706X

Budke, C. M. (2006). Global socioeconomic impact of cystic echinococcosis. *Emerg Infect Dis*, Vol.12, No.2), pp. 296-303, ISSN: 1080-6040

Cabrera, P. A., Irabedra, P., Orlando, D., Rista, L., Haran, G., Vinals, G., Blanco, M. T., Alvarez, M., Elola, S., Morosoli, D., Morana, A., Bondad, M., Sambran, Y., Heinzen, T., Chans, L., Pineyro, L., Perez, D. &Pereyra, I. (2003). National prevalence of larval echinococcosis in sheep in slaughtering plants Ovis aries as an indicator in control programmes in Uruguay. *Acta Trop*, Vol.85, No.2, pp. 281-285, ISSN: 0001-706X

Chai, J., Sultan, Y. &Wei, M. (1989). An investigation on the epidemiologic baseline of hydatid disease in Xinjiang, China. I. A sero-epidemiological survey of human hydatidosis. *Endemic Disease Bulletin (in Chinese)*, Vol.4, pp. 1-8, ISSN: 1000-3711

Chamekh, M., Gras-Masse, H., Bossus, M., Facon, B., Dissous, C., Tartar, A. &Capron, A. (1992). Diagnostic value of a synthetic peptide derived from *Echinococcus granulosus* recombinant protein. *J Clin Invest*, Vol.89, No.2, pp. 458-464, ISSN: 0021-9738

Chemale, G., Ferreira, H. B., Barrett, J., Brophy, P. M. &Zaha, A. (2005). *Echinococcus granulosus* antigen B hydrophobic ligand binding properties. *Biochim Biophys Acta*, Vol.1747, No.2, pp.189-194, ISSN: 0006-3002

Chemale, G., Haag, K. L., Ferreira, H. B. &Zaha, A. (2001). *Echinococcus granulosus* antigen B is encoded by a gene family. *Mol Biochem* Parasitol, Vol.116, No.2, pp. 233-237, ISSN: 0166-6851

Chi, P. S., Fan, Y. L., Zhang, W. B., Zhang, Z. Z., Alili, H. &Zhang, Y. L. (1989). The epidemic situations of cystic echinococcosis in China. *Xinjiang Agricultural Sciences* 1989, Vol.3, pp. 35-38(*in Chinese*), ISSN: 1001-4330

Clutterbuck, E. J., Hirst, E. M. &Sanderson, C. J. (1989). Human interleukin-5 (IL-5) regulates the production of eosinophils in human bone marrow cultures: comparison and interaction with IL-1, IL-3, IL-6, and GMCSF. *Blood,* Vol.73, No.6, pp.1504-1512, ISSN: 0006-4971

Collaboration, groups, in &China (2005). A national survey on current status of the important parasitic diseases in human population. *Zhongguo Ji Sheng Chong Xue Yu Ji Sheng Chong Bing Za Zhi,* Vol.23, pp. 332-340, ISSN: 1000-7423

Craig, P. (1997). Immunodiagnosis of Echinococcus granulosus and comparison of techniques for diagnosis of canine echinococcosis. In: *Compendium on echinococcosis in Africa and Middle Eastern counties with special reference to Morocco,* F.L. Andersen, J.J. Chai, F.J. Liu (Eds.), 85-118, Provo, Utah: Brigham Young University,

Craig, P. S. (1986). Detection of specific circulating antigen, immune complexes and antibodies in human hydatidosis from Turkana (Kenya) and Great Britain, by enzyme-immunoassay. *Parasite Immunol,* Vol. 8, No.2, pp. 171-188, ISSN: 1365-3024

Craig, P. S. (1993). *Immunodiagnosis of Echinococcus granulosus.* Provo, Utah: Brigham Young University.

Craig, P. S. &Larrieu, E. (2006). Control of cystic echinococcosis/hydatidosis: 1863-2002. *Adv Parasitol,* Vol.61, pp. 443-508, ISSN: 0065-308X

Craig, P. S., McManus, D. P., Lightowlers, M. W., Chabalgoity, J. A., Garcia, H. H., Gavidia, C. M., Gilman, R. H., Gonzalez, A. E., Lorca, M., Naquira, C., Nieto, A. &Schantz, P. M. (2007). Prevention and control of cystic echinococcosis. *Lancet Infect Dis,* Vol.7, No.6, pp. 385-394, ISSN: 1473-3099

Craig, P. S., Mitchell, G. F., Cruise, K. M. &Rickard, M. D. (1980). Hybridoma antibody immunoassays for the detection of parasitic infection: attempts to produce an immunodiagnostic reagent for a larval taeniid cestode infection. *Aust J Exp Biol Med Sci,* Vol.58, No.4, pp. 339-350, ISSN: 0004-945X

Craig, P. S. &Nelson, G. S. (1984). The detection of circulating antigen in human hydatid disease. *Ann Trop Med Parasitol,* Vol.78, No.3, pp. 219-227, ISSN: 1364-8594

Craig, P. S. &Rickard, M. D. (1982). Antibody responses of experimentally infected lambs to antigens collected during in vitro maintenance of the adult, metacestode or oncosphere stages of *Taenia hydatigena* and *Taenia ovis* with further observations on anti-oncospheral antibodies. *Z Parasitenkd,* Vol.67, No.2, pp. 197-209, ISSN: 0044-3255

Craig, P. S., Zeyhle, E. &Romig, T. (1986). Hydatid disease: research and control in Turkana. II. The role of immunological techniques for the diagnosis of hydatid disease. *Trans R Soc Trop Med Hyg,* Vol.80, No.2, pp. 183-192, ISSN: 0035-9203

Daeki, A. O., Craig, P. S. &Shambesh, M. K. (2000). IgG-subclass antibody responses and the natural history of hepatic cystic echinococcosis in asymptomatic patients. *Ann Trop Med Parasitol,* Vol.94, No.4, pp. 319-328, ISSN: 1364-8594

Dai, W. J., Hemphill, A., Waldvogel, A., Ingold, K., Deplazes, P., Mossmann, H. &Gottstein, B. (2001). Major carbohydrate antigen of *Echinococcus multilocularis* induces an immunoglobulin G response independent of alphabeta+ CD4+ T cells. *Infect Immun,* Vol.69, No.10, pp. 6074-6083, ***ISSN***: 0019-9567

de la Rue, M. L., Yamano, K., Almeida, C. E., Iesbich, M. P., Fernandes, C. D., Goto, A., Kouguchi, H. &Takahashi, K. (2010). Serological reactivity of patients with

Echinococcus infections (*E. granulosus*, *E. vogeli*, and *E. multilocularis*) against three antigen B subunits. *Parasitol Res*, Vol.106, No.3, pp. 741-745, ISSN:0932-0113

Delunardo, F., Ortona, E., Margutti, P., Perdicchio, M., Vacirca, D., Teggi, A., Sorice, M. &Siracusano, A. (2010). Identification of a novel 19 kDa *Echinococcus granulosus* antigen. *Acta Trop*, Vol.113, No.1, pp.42-47, ISSN: 0001-706X

Deplazes, P. (2006). Ecology and epidemiology of *Echinococcus multilocularis* in Europe. *Parassitologia*, Vol.48, No.1-2, pp. 37-39, ISSN: 0048-2951

Dessaint, J. P., Bout, D., Wattre, P. &Capron, A. (1975). Quantitative determination of specific IgE antibodies to *Echinococcus granulosus* and IgE levels in sera from patients with hydatid disease. *Immunology*, Vol.29, No.5, pp. 813-823, ISSN: 1365-2567

Dvoroznakova, E., Hrckova, G., Boroskova, Z., Velebny, S. &Dubinsky, P. (2004). Effect of treatment with free and liposomized albendazole on selected immunological parameters and cyst growth in mice infected with *Echinococcus multilocularis*. *Parasitol Int*, Vol.53, No.4, pp. 315-325, ISSN: 1383-5769

Eckert, J., Conraths, F. J. &Tackmann, K. (2000). Echinococcosis: an emerging or re-emerging zoonosis? *Int J Parasitol*, Vol.30, No.12-13, pp. 1283-1294, ISSN: 0020-7519

Emery, I., Liance, M. &Leclerc, C. (1997). Secondary *Echinococcus multilocularis* infection in A/J mice: delayed metacestode development is associated with Th1 cytokine production. *Parasite Immunol*, Vol.19, No.11, pp. 493-503, ISSN: 1365-3024

Feng, X., Wen, H., Zhang, Z., Chen, X., Ma, X., Zhang, J., Qi, X., Bradshaw, H., Vuitton, D. &Craig, P. S. (2010). Dot immunogold filtration assay (DIGFA) with multiple native antigens for rapid serodiagnosis of human cystic and alveolar echinococcosis. *Acta Trop*, Vol.113, No.2, pp. 114-120, ISSN: 1873-6254

Fernandez, V., Ferreira, H. B., Fernandez, C., Zaha, A. &Nieto, A. (1996). Molecular characterisation of a novel 8-kDa subunit of *Echinococcus granulosus* antigen B. *Mol Biochem Parasitol*, Vol.77, No.2, pp. 247-250, ISSN: 0166-6851

Force, L., Torres, J. M., Carrillo, A. &Busca, J. (1992). Evaluation of eight serological tests in the diagnosis of human echinococcosis and follow-up. *Clin Infect Dis*, Vol.15, No.3, pp. 473-480, ISSN: 1537-6591

Frosch, P. M., Geier, C., Kaup, F. J., Muller, A. &Frosch, M. (1993). Molecular cloning of an echinococcal microtrichal antigen immunoreactive in *Echinococcus multilocularis* disease. *Mol Biochem Parasitol*, Vol. 58, No.2, pp. 301-310, ISSN: 0166-6851

Fujimoto, Y., Ito, A., Ishikawa, Y., Inoue, M., Suzuki, Y., Ohhira, M., Ohtake, T. &Kohgo, Y. (2005). Usefulness of recombinant Em18-ELISA to evaluate efficacy of treatment in patients with alveolar echinococcosis. *J Gastroenterol*, Vol.40, No.4, pp. 426-431, ISSN: 1435-5922

Gatti, A., Alvarez, A. R., Araya, D., Mancini, S., Herrero, E., Santillan, G. &Larrieu, E. (2007). Ovine echinococcosis I. Immunological diagnosis by enzyme immunoassay. *Vet Parasitol*, Vol.143, No.2, pp. 112-121, ISSN: 0304-4017

Gavidia, C. M., Gonzalez, A. E., Zhang, W., McManus, D. P., Lopera, L., Ninaquispe, B., Garcia, H. H., Rodriguez, S., Verastegui, M., Calderon, C., Pan, W. K. &Gilman, R. H. (2008). Diagnosis of cystic echinococcosis, central Peruvian Highlands. *Emerg Infect Dis*, Vol.14, No.2, pp. 260-266, ISSN: 1080-6040

Ghorbanpoor, M., Razi Jalali, M. H., Hoghooghi Rad, N., Nabavi, L., Esmail Zadeh, S., Rafiei, A. &Haji Hajikolaei, M. R. (2006). Detection of specific hydatid antigens and antibodies in serum and urine of experimentally infected sheep. *Vet Parasitol*, Vol.142, No.1-2, pp. 91-94 ISSN: 0304-4017

Godot, V., Harraga, S., Beurton, I., Deschaseaux, M., Sarciron, E., Gottstein, B. &Vuitton, D. A. (2000). Resistance/susceptibility to *Echinococcus multilocularis* infection and cytokine profile in humans. I. Comparison of patients with progressive and abortive lesions. *Clin Exp Immunol*, Vol.121, No.3, pp. 484-490, ISSN: 1474-1741

Gonzalez-Sapienza, G., Lorenzo, C. &Nieto, A. (2000). Improved immunodiagnosis of cystic hydatid disease by using a synthetic peptide with higher diagnostic value than that of its parent protein, *Echinococcus granulosus* antigen B. *J Clin Microbiol*, Vol.38, No.11, pp. 3979-3983, ISSN: 1098-660X

Gonzalez, G., Spinelli, P., Lorenzo, C., Hellman, U., Nieto, A., Willis, A. &Salinas, G. (2000). Molecular characterization of P-29, a metacestode-specific component of *Echinococcus granulosus* which is immunologically related to, but distinct from, antigen 5. *Mol Biochem Parasitol*, Vol.105, No.2), pp. 177-184, ISSN: 0166-6851

Gottstein, B. (1984). An immunoassay for the detection of circulating antigens in human echinococcosis. *Am J Trop Med Hyg*, Vol.33, No.6, pp. 1185-1191, ISSN: 0002-9637

Gottstein, B. (1985). Purification and characterization of a specific antigen from *Echinococcus multilocularis*. *Parasite Immunol*, Vol.7, No.3, pp. 201-212, ISSN: 1365-3024

Gottstein, B., Dai, W. J., Walker, M., Stettler, M., Muller, N. &Hemphill, A. (2002). An intact laminated layer is important for the establishment of secondary *Echinococcus multilocularis* infection. *Parasitol Res*, Vol.88, No.9, pp. 822-828, ISSN:0932-0113

Gottstein, B. &Felleisen, R. (1995). Protective immune mechanisms against the metacestode of *Echinococcus multilocularis*. *Parasitol Today*, Vol.11, No.9, pp. 320-326, ISSN: 0169-4758

Gottstein, B., Jacquier, P., Bresson-Hadni, S. &Eckert, J. (1993). Improved primary immunodiagnosis of alveolar echinococcosis in humans by an enzyme-linked immunosorbent assay using the Em2plus antigen. *J Clin Microbiol*, Vol.31, No.2, pp. 373-376, ISSN: 1098-660X

Gottstein, B., Wittwer, M., Schild, M., Merli, M., Leib, S. L., Muller, N., Muller, J. &Jaggi, R. (2010). Hepatic gene expression profile in mice perorally infected with *Echinococcus multilocularis* eggs. *PLoS One*, Vol.5, No.4, pp. e9779, ISSN: 1932-6203

Haag, K. L., Gottstein, B., Muller, N., Schnorr, A. &Ayala, F. J. (2006). Redundancy and recombination in the *Echinococcus* AgB multigene family: is there any similarity with protozoan contingency genes? *Parasitology*, Vol.133, (Pt. 4), pp.411-419, ISSN: 0031-1820

Harraga, S., Godot, V., Bresson-Hadni, S., Mantion, G. &Vuitton, D. A. (2003). Profile of cytokine production within the periparasitic granuloma in human alveolar echinococcosis. *Acta Trop*, Vol85, No.2, pp. 231-236, ISSN: 0001-706X

Harrison, L. J., Joshua, G. W., Wright, S. H. &Parkhouse, R. M. (1989). Specific detection of circulating surface/secreted glycoproteins of viable cysticerci in *Taenia saginata* cysticercosis. *Parasite Immunol*, Vol.11, No.4, pp. 351-370, ISSN: 1365-3024

Hegglin, D., Bontadina, F., Gloor, S., Romig, T., Deplazes, P. &Kern, P. (2008). Survey of public knowledge about *Echinococcus multilocularis* in four European countries: need for proactive information. *BMC Public Health* Vol. 8: 247-257, ISSN:1471-2458

Helbig, M., Frosch, P., Kern, P. &Frosch, M. (1993). Serological differentiation between cystic and alveolar echinococcosis by use of recombinant larval antigens. *J Clin Microbiol*, Vol.31, No.12, pp. 3211-3215, ISSN: 1098-660X

Hernandez-Gonzalez, A., Muro, A., Barrera, I., Ramos, G., Orduna, A. & Siles-Lucas, M. (2008). Usefulness of four different *Echinococcus granulosus* recombinant antigens for serodiagnosis of unilocular hydatid disease (UHD) and postsurgical follow-up of patients treated for UHD. *Clin Vaccine Immunol*, Vol.15, No.1, pp. 147-153, ISSN: 1556-679X

Ibrahem, M. M., Craig, P. S., McVie, A., Ersfeld, K. &Rogan, M. T. (1996). *Echinococcus granulosus* antigen B and seroreactivity in natural ovine hydatidosis. *Res Vet Sci*, Vol.61, No.2, pp. 102-106, ISSN: 0034-5288

Irabuena, O., Nieto, A., Ferreira, A. M., Battistoni, J. &Ferragut, G. (2000). Characterization and optimization of bovine *Echinococcus granulosus* cyst fluid to be used in immunodiagnosis of hydatid disease by ELISA. *Rev Inst Med Trop Sao Paulo*, Vol.42, No.5, pp. 255-262, ISSN 0036-4665

Ito, A., Ma, L., Schantz, P. M., Gottstein, B., Liu, Y. H., Chai, J. J., Abdel-Hafez, S. K., Altintas, N., Joshi, D. D., Lightowlers, M. W. &Pawlowski, Z. S. (1999). Differential serodiagnosis for cystic and alveolar echinococcosis using fractions of *Echinococcus granulosus* cyst fluid (antigen B) and *E. multilocularis* protoscolex (EM18). *Am J Trop Med Hyg*, Vol.60, No.2, pp. 188-192, ISSN: 0002-9637

Ito, A., Sako, Y., Yamasaki, H., Mamuti, W., Nakaya, K., Nakao, M. &Ishikawa, Y. (2003a). Development of Em18-immunoblot and Em18-ELISA for specific diagnosis of alveolar echinococcosis. *Acta Trop*, Vol.85, No.2, pp. 173-182, ISSN: 0001-706X

Ito, A., Urbani, C., Jiamin, Q., Vuitton, D. A., Dongchuan, Q., Heath, D. D., Craig, P. S., Zheng, F. &Schantz, P. M. (2003b). Control of echinococcosis and cysticercosis: a public health challenge to international cooperation in China. *Acta Trop*, Vol.86, No.1, pp. 3-17, ISSN: 0001-706X

Jiang, L., Wen, H. &Ito, A. (2001). Immunodiagnostic differentiation of alveolar and cystic echinococcosis using ELISA test with 18-kDa antigen extracted from *Echinococcus* protoscoleces. *Trans R Soc Trop Med Hyg*, Vol.95, No.3, pp. 285-288, ISSN: 0035-9203

Kalantari, E., Bandehpour, M., Pazoki, R., Taghipoor-Lailabadi, N., Khazan, H., Mosaffa, N., Nazaripouya, M. R. &Kazemi, B. (2010). Application of recombinant *Echinococcus granulosua* antigen B to ELISA kits for diagnosing hydatidosis. *Parasitol Res*, Vol.106, No.4, pp. 847-851, ISSN:0932-0113

Kamenetzky, L., Muzulin, P. M., Gutierrez, A. M., Angel, S. O., Zaha, A., Guarnera, E. A. &Rosenzvit, M. C. (2005). High polymorphism in genes encoding antigen B from human infecting strains of *Echinococcus granulosus*. *Parasitology*, Vol.131, (Pt 6), pp.805-815, ISSN: 0031-1820

Kanan, J. H. &Chain, B. M. (2006). Modulation of dendritic cell differentiation and cytokine secretion by the hydatid cyst fluid of *Echinococcus granulosus*. *Immunology*, Vol.118, No.2), pp. 271-278, ISSN: 1365-2567

Kanwar, J. R. &Kanwar, R. (1994). Purification and partial immunochemical characterization of a low molecular mass, diagnostic *Echinococcus granulosus* immunogen for sheep hydatidosis. *FEMS Immunol Med Microbiol*, Vol.9, No.2, pp. 101-107, ISSN: 0928-8244

Kanwar, J. R., Kanwar, R. K., Grewal, A. S. &Vinayak, V. K. (1994). Significance of detection of immune-complexed 8 kDa hydatid-specific antigen for immunodiagnosis of hydatidosis. *FEMS Immunol Med Microbiol*, Vol.9, No.3, pp. 231-236, ISSN: 0928-8244

Khabiri, A. R., Bagheri, F., Assmar, M. &Siavashi, M. R. (2006). Analysis of specific IgE and IgG subclass antibodies for diagnosis of *Echinococcus granulosus*. *Parasite Immunol*, Vol.28, No.8, pp. 357-362, ISSN: 1365-3024

King, C. L. &Nutman, T. B. (1993). IgE and IgG subclass regulation by IL-4 and IFN-gamma in human helminth infections. Assessment by B cell precursor frequencies. *J Immunol*, Vol.151, No.1, pp. 458-465, ***ISSN***: 1550-6606

Kittelberger, R., Reichel, M. P., Jenner, J., Heath, D. D., Lightowlers, M. W., Moro, P., Ibrahem, M. M., Craig, P. S. &O'Keefe, J. S. (2002). Evaluation of three enzyme-linked immunosorbent assays (ELISAs) for the detection of serum antibodies in sheep infected with *Echinococcus granulosus*. *Vet Parasitol*, Vol.110, No.1-2, pp. 57-76, ISSN: 0304-4017

Kocherscheidt, L., Flakowski, A. K., Gruner, B., Hamm, D. M., Dietz, K., Kern, P. &Soboslay, P. T. (2008). *Echinococcus multilocularis*: inflammatory and regulatory chemokine responses in patients with progressive, stable and cured alveolar echinococcosis. *Exp Parasitol*, Vol.119, No.4, pp. 467-474, ISSN: 0014-4894

Korkmaz, M., Inceboz, T., Celebi, F., Babaoglu, A. &Uner, A. (2004). Use of two sensitive and specific immunoblot markers, em70 and em90, for diagnosis of alveolar echinococcosis. *J Clin Microbiol*, Vol.42, No.7, pp. 3350-3352, ISSN: 1098-660X

Larrieu, E., Costa, M. T., Cantoni, G., Alvarez, R., Cavagion, L., Labanchi, J. L., Bigatti, R., Araya, D., Herrero, E., Alvarez, E., Mancini, S. &Cabrera, P. (2001). Ovine *Echinococcus granulosus* transmission dynamics in the province of Rio Negro, Argentina, 1980-1999. *Vet Parasitol*, Vol.98, No.4, pp. 263-272, ISSN: 0304-4017

Leggatt, G. R. &McManus, D. P. (1994). Identification and diagnostic value of a major antibody epitope on the 12 kDa antigen from *Echinococcus granulosus* (hydatid disease) cyst fluid. *Parasite Immunol*, Vol.16, No.2, pp. 87-96, ISSN: 1365-3024

Li, F. R., Shi, Y. E., Shi, D. Z., Vuitton, D. A. &Craig, P. S. (2003a). [Kinetic analysis of cytokines and immunoglobulin G subclass in BALB/c mice infected with *Echinococcus* alveolaris]. *Zhongguo Ji Sheng Chong Xue Yu Ji Sheng Chong Bing Za Zhi*, Vol.21, No.6, pp.357-360, ISSN: 1000-7423

Li, J., Zhang, W. B. &McManus, D. P. (2004). Recombinant antigens for immunodiagnosis of cystic echinococcosis. *Biol Proced Online*, Vol.6, pp. 67-77,

Li, J., Zhang, W. B., Wilson, M., Ito, A. &McManus, D. P. (2003b). A novel recombinant antigen for immunodiagnosis of human cystic echinococcosis. *Journal of infectious diseases*, Vol.188, No.12, pp. 1952-1961,

Li, T., Ito, A., Chen, X., Sako, Y., Qiu, J., Xiao, N., Qiu, D., Nakao, M., Yanagida, T. &Craig, P. S. (2010). Specific IgG responses to recombinant antigen B and em18 in cystic and alveolar echinococcosis in china. *Clin Vaccine Immunol*, Vol.17, No.3, pp. 470-475,

Li, T. Y., Qiu, J. M., Yang, W., Craig, P. S., Chen, X. W., Xiao, N., Ito, A., Giraudoux, P., Mamuti, W., Yu, W. &Schantz, P. M. (2005). Echinococcosis in Tibetan populations, western Sichuan Province, China. *Emerg Infect Dis*, Vol.11, No.12, pp. 1866-1873, ISSN: 1080-6040

Lightowlers, M. W. (1990). Cestode infections in animals: immunological diagnosis and vaccination. *Rev Sci Tech*, Vol.9, No.2, pp. 463-487,

Lightowlers, M. W. &Gottstein, B. (1995). *Echinococcosis/hydatidosis: antigens, immunological and molecular diagnosis.* Wallingford, Oxon, UK: CAB International,

Lightowlers, M. W., Liu, D. Y., Haralambous, A. &Rickard, M. D. (1989). Subunit composition and specificity of the major cyst fluid antigens of *Echinococcus granulosus. Mol Biochem Parasitol*, Vol.37, No.2, pp. 171-182, ISSN: 0166-6851

Lightowlers, M. W., Rickard, M. D., Honey, R. D., Obendorf, D. L. &Mitchell, G. F. (1984). Serological diagnosis of *Echinococcus granulosus* infection in sheep using cyst fluid antigen processed by antibody affinity chromatography. *Aust Vet J*, Vol.61, No.4, pp. 101-108,

Liu, D., Rickard, M. D. &Lightowlers, M. W. (1993). Assessment of monoclonal antibodies to *Echinococcus granulosus* antigen 5 and antigen B for detection of human hydatid circulating antigens. *Parasitology*, Vol. 106, (Pt 1), pp. 75-81, ISSN: 0031-1820

Lorenzo, C., Ferreira, H. B., Monteiro, K. M., Rosenzvit, M., Kamenetzky, L., Garcia, H. H., Vasquez, Y., Naquira, C., Sanchez, E., Lorca, M., Contreras, M., Last, J. A. &Gonzalez-Sapienza, G. G. (2005a). Comparative analysis of the diagnostic performance of six major *Echinococcus granulosus* antigens assessed in a double-blind, randomized multicenter study. *J Clin Microbiol*, Vol.43, No.6, pp. 2764-2770, ISSN: 1098-660X

Lorenzo, C., Last, J. A. &Gonzalez-Sapienza, G. G. (2005b). The immunogenicity of *Echinococcus granulosus* antigen 5 is determined by its post-translational modifications. *Parasitology*, Vol.131, (Pt 5), pp. 669-677, ISSN: 0031-1820

Lv, G. D., Liu, T., Lin, R. Y., Wang, X., Wang, J. H., Ren, Z. H., Wen, H. &Lu, X. M. (2009). Immunoreactivity of the recombinant protein of *Echinococcus granulosus* antigen B. *Zhongguo Ji Sheng Chong Xue Yu Ji Sheng Chong Bing Za Zhi*, Vol.27, No.2, pp. 107-110, ISSN: 1000-7423

Macpherson, C. N., Kachani, M., Lyagoubi, M., Berrada, M., Shepherd, M., Fields, P. F. &El Hasnaoui, M. (2004). Cystic echinococcosis in the Berber of the Mid Atlas mountains, Morocco: new insights into the natural history of the disease in humans. *Ann Trop Med Parasitol*, Vol.98, No.5, pp. 481-490, ISSN: 1364-8594

Magambo, J. K., Zeyhle, Wachira, T. M., Wachira, J. &Raasen, T. (1995). Cellular immunity to *Echinococcus granulosus* cysts. *Afr J Health Sci*, Vol.2, No.1, pp. 250-253, ISSN: 1478-2642

Mahmoud, M. S. &Abou Gamra, M. M. (2004). Alkaline phosphatase from *Echinococcus granulosus* metacestodes for immunodiagnosis of human cystic echinococcosis. *J Egypt Soc Parasitol*, Vol.34, No.3, pp. 865-879, ISSN: 0253-5890

Mamuti, W., Sako, Y., Bart, J. M., Nakao, M., Ma, X., Wen, H. &Ito, A. (2007). Molecular characterization of a novel gene encoding an 8-kDa-subunit of antigen B from *Echinococcus granulosus* genotypes 1 and 6. *Parasitol Int.*, Vol.56, No.4, pp. 313-316, ISSN: 1383-5769

Manfras, B. J., Reuter, S., Wendland, T. &Kern, P. (2002). Increased activation and oligoclonality of peripheral CD8(+) T cells in the chronic human helminth infection alveolar echinococcosis. *Infect Immun*, Vol.70, No.3, pp. 1168-1174, *ISSN*: 0019-9567

Margos, M. C., Grandgirard, D., Leib, S. &Gottstein, B. (2011). In vitro induction of lymph node cell proliferation by mouse bone marrow dendritic cells following stimulation with different *Echinococcus multilocularis* antigens. *J Helminthol*, Vol.85, No.02, pp. 128-137, ISSN: 1475-2697

Marinova, I., Nikolov, G., Michova, A., Kurdova, R. &Petrunov, B. (2011). Quantitative assessment of serum-specific IgE in the diagnosis of human cystic echinococcosis. *Parasite Immunol*, Vol.33, No.7, pp. 371–376, ISSN: 1365-3024

Matossian, R. M., Awar, G. N., Radwan, H., Craig, P. S. &Meshefedjian, G. A. (1992). Immune status during albendazole therapy for hydatidosis. *Ann Trop Med Parasitol*, Vol.86, No.1, pp. 67-75, ISSN: 1364-8594

Matsumoto, J., Kouguchi, H., Oku, Y. &Yagi, K. (2010). Primary alveolar echinococcosis: course of larval development and antibody responses in intermediate host rodents with different genetic backgrounds after oral infection with eggs of *Echinococcus multilocularis*. *Parasitol Int*, Vol.59, No.3, pp. 435-444, ISSN: 1383-5769

Matsumoto, J., Yagi, K., Nonaka, N., Oku, Y. &Kamiya, M. (1998). Time-course of antibody response in mice against oral infection with eggs of *Echinococcus multilocularis*. *Parasitology*, Vol.116, (Pt 5), pp. 463-469, ISSN: 0031-1820

McManus, D. P. (2006). Molecular discrimination of taeniid cestodes. *Parasitol Int* 55 Suppl: S31-37, ISSN: 1383-5769

McManus, D. P. &Thompson, R. C. (2003). Molecular epidemiology of cystic echinococcosis. *Parasitology*, Vol.127 Suppl: S37-51, ISSN: 0031-1820

McManus, D. P., Zhang, W., Li, J. &Bartley, P. B. (2003). Echinococcosis. *Lancet*, Vol.362, No.9392, pp. 1295-1304,

McVie, A., Ersfeld, K., Rogan, M. T. &Craig, P. S. (1997). Expression and immunological characterisation of *Echinococcus granulosus* recombinant antigen B for IgG4 subclass detection in human cystic echinococcosis. *Acta Trop*, Vol.67, No.1-2, pp. 19-35, ISSN: 0001-706X

Mejri, N., Muller, J. &Gottstein, B. (2011a). Intraperitoneal murine *Echinococcus multilocularis* infection induces differentiation of TGF-beta expressing DCs that remain immature. *Parasite Immunol*, Vol.33, No.9, pp. 471-482, ISSN: 1365-3024

Mejri, N., Muller, N., Hemphill, A. &Gottstein, B. (2011b). Intraperitoneal *Echinococcus multilocularis* infection in mice modulates peritoneal CD4+ and CD8+ regulatory T cell development. *Parasitol Int*, Vol.60, No.1, pp. 45-53, ISSN: 1383-5769

Mezioug, D. &Touil-Boukoffa, C. (2009). Cytokine profile in human hydatidosis: possible role in the immunosurveillance of patients infected with *Echinococcus granulosus*. *Parasite*, Vol.16, No.1, pp. 57-64, ISSN 1252-607X

Moore, K. W., de Waal Malefyt, R., Coffman, R. L. &O'Garra, A. (2001). Interleukin-10 and the interleukin-10 receptor. *Annu Rev Immunol*, Vol.19, pp. 683-765, ISSN: 0732-0582

Moosa, R. A. &Abdel-Hafez, S. K. (1994). Serodiagnosis and seroepidemiology of human unilocular hydatidosis in Jordan. *Parasitol Res*, Vol.80, No.8, pp. 664-671, ISSN:0932-0113

Moro, P. L., Garcia, H. H., Gonzales, A. E., Bonilla, J. J., Verastegui, M. &Gilman, R. H. (2005). Screening for cystic echinococcosis in an endemic region of Peru using portable ultrasonography and the enzyme-linked immunoelectrotransfer blot (EITB) assay. *Parasitol Res*, Vol.96, No.4, pp. 242-246, ISSN:0932-0113

Moro, P. L., McDonald, J., Gilman, R. H., Silva, B., Verastegui, M., Malqui, V., Lescano, G., Falcon, N., Montes, G. &Bazalar, H. (1997). Epidemiology of *Echinococcus granulosus* infection in the central Peruvian Andes. *Bull World Health Organ*, Vol.75, No.6, pp. 553-561, ISSN:0042-9686

Muller, N., Frei, E., Nunez, S. &Gottstein, B. (2007). Improved serodiagnosis of alveolar echinococcosis of humans using an in vitro-produced *Echinococcus multilocularis* antigen. *Parasitology*, Vol.134, (Pt 6), pp. 879-888, ISSN: 0031-1820

Myjak, P., Nahorski, W., Pietkiewicz, H., von Nickisch-Rosenegk, M., Stolarczyk, J., Kacprzak, E., Felczak-Korzybska, I., Szostakowska, B. &Lucius, R. (2003). Molecular confirmation of human alveolar echinococcosis in Poland. *Clin Infect Dis* Vol. 37, No. 8, e121-125, ISSN:1537-6591

Nasrieh, M. A. &Abdel-Hafez, S. K. (2004). *Echinococcus granulosus* in Jordan: assessment of various antigenic preparations for use in the serodiagnosis of surgically confirmed cases using enzyme immuno assays and the indirect haemagglutination test. *Diagn Microbiol Infect Dis*, Vol.48, No.2, pp. 117-123, ISSN: 0732-8893

Onyango-Abuje, J. A., Nginyi, J. M., Rugutt, M. K., Wright, S. H., Lumumba, P., Hughes, G. &Harrison, L. J. (1996). Seroepidemiological survey of *Taenia saginata* cysticercosis in Kenya. *Vet Parasitol*, Vol.64, No.3, pp. 177-185, ISSN: 0304-4017

Ortona, E., Margutti, P., Delunardo, F., Nobili, V., Profumo, E., Rigano, R., Buttari, B., Carulli, G., Azzara, A., Teggi, A., Bruschi, F. &Siracusano, A. (2005). Screening of an *Echinococcus granulosus* cDNA library with IgG4 from patients with cystic echinococcosis identifies a new tegumental protein involved in the immune escape. *Clin Exp Immunol*, Vol.142, No.3, pp. 528-538, ISSN: 1474-1741

Ortona, E., Rigano, R., Margutti, P., Notargiacomo, S., Ioppolo, S., Vaccari, S., Barca, S., Buttari, B., Profumo, E., Teggi, A. &Siracusano, A. (2000). Native and recombinant antigens in the immunodiagnosis of human cystic echinococcosis. *Parasite Immunol*, Vol.22, No.11, pp. 553-559, ISSN: 1365-3024

Pawlowski, Z. S., Eckert, J., Vuitton, D. A., Ammann, R. W., Kern, P., Craig, P. S., Dar, F. K., De Rosa, F., Filice, C., Gottstein, B., Grimm, F., Macpherson, C. N. L., Sato, N., Todorov, T., Uchino, J., von Sinner, W. &Wen, H. (2001). Echinococcosis in humans: clinical aspects, diagnosis and treatment, In: *WHO/OIE Manual on Echinococcosis in Humans and Animals: a Public Health Problem of Global Concern*, J. Eckert, M. A. Gemmell, F.-X. Mesli and Z. S. Pawlowski (Eds.) World Organisation for Animal Health and World Health Organisation, ISBN 92-9044-522-X, Paris, France.

Pearce, E. J. &MacDonald, A. S. (2002). The immunobiology of schistosomiasis. *Nat Rev Immunol*, Vol.2, No.7, pp. 499-511, ISSN: 1474-1733

Peng, X., Li, J., Wu, X., Zhang, S., Niu, J., Chen, X., Yao, J. &Sun, H. (2006). Detection of Osteopontin in the pericyst of human hepatic *Echinococcus granulosus*. *Acta Trop*, Vol.100, No.3, pp. 163-171, ISSN: 0001-706X

Petrova, R. F. (1968). Blood picture in experimental hydatidosis in sheep › *Materiali Seminara-Soveshch. Borbe Gel'mint. Zhivot. Chimk. Alma-Ala*, pp. *115-116 (in Russian)*.

Pinon, J. M., Poirriez, J., Lepan, H., Geers, R., Penna, R. &Fernandez, D. (1987). Value of isotypic characterization of antibodies to *Echinococcus granulosus* by enzyme-linked immuno-filtration assay. *Eur J Clin Microbiol*, Vol.6, No.3, pp. 291-295, ISSN: 0934-9723

Poretti, D., Felleisen, E., Grimm, F., Pfister, M., Teuscher, F., Zuercher, C., Reichen, J. &Gottstein, B. (1999). Differential immunodiagnosis between cystic hydatid disease and other cross-reactive pathologies. *Am J Trop Med Hyg*, Vol.60, No.2, pp. 193-198, ISSN: 0002-9637

Ravinder, P. T., Parija, S. C. &Rao, K. S. (1997). Evaluation of human hydatid disease before and after surgery and chemotherapy by demonstration of hydatid antigens and antibodies in serum. *J Med Microbiol*, Vol.46, No.10, pp. 859-864, ISSN: 0022-2615

Ravinder, P. T., Parija, S. C. &Rao, K. S. (2000). Urinary hydatid antigen detection by coagglutination, a cost-effective and rapid test for diagnosis of cystic echinococcosis in a rural or field setting. *J Clin Microbiol*, Vol.38, No.8, pp. 2972-2974, ISSN: 1098-660X

Read, A. J., Casey, J. L., Coley, A. M., Foley, M., Gauci, C. G., Jackson, D. C. &Lightowlers, M. W. (2009). Isolation of antibodies specific to a single conformation-dependant antigenic determinant on the EG95 hydatid vaccine. *Vaccine*, Vol.27, No.7, pp. 1024-1031, ISSN: 0264-410X

Reiter-Owona, I., Gruner, B., Frosch, M., Hoerauf, A., Kern, P. &Tappe, D. (2009). Serological confirmatory testing of alveolar and cystic echinococcosis in clinical practice: results of a comparative study with commercialized and in-house assays. *Clin Lab*, Vol.55, No.1-2, pp. 41-48, ISSN: 1433-6510

Rickard, M. D. (1984). Serological diagnosis and post-operative surveillance of human hydatid disease. I. Latex agglutination and immunoelectrophoresis using crude cyst fluid antigen. *Pathology*, Vol.16, No.2, pp. 207-210, ISSN: 0172-8113

Rickard, M. D., Honey, R. D., Brumley, J. L. &Mitchell, G. F. (1984). Serological diagnosis and post-operative surveillance of human hydatid disease. II. The enzyme-linked immunosorbent assay (ELISA) using various antigens. *Pathology*, Vol.16, No.2, pp. 211-215, ISSN: 0172-8113

Rigano, R., Buttari, B., De Falco, E., Profumo, E., Ortona, E., Margutti, P., Scotta, C., Teggi, A. &Siracusano, A. (2004). *Echinococcus granulosus*-specific T-cell lines derived from patients at various clinical stages of cystic echinococcosis. *Parasite Immunol*, Vol.26, No.1, pp. 45-52, ISSN: 1365-3024

Rigano, R., Buttari, B., Profumo, E., Ortona, E., Delunardo, F., Margutti, P., Mattei, V., Teggi, A., Sorice, M. &Siracusano, A. (2007). *Echinococcus granulosus* antigen B impairs human dendritic cell differentiation and polarizes immature dendritic cell maturation towards a Th2 cell response. *Infect Immun*, Vol.75, No.4, pp. 1667-1678, ***ISSN***: 0019-9567

Rigano, R., Profumo, E., Bruschi, F., Carulli, G., Azzara, A., Ioppolo, S., Buttari, B., Ortona, E., Margutti, P., Teggi, A. &Siracusano, A. (2001). Modulation of human immune response by *Echinococcus granulosus* antigen B and its possible role in evading host defenses. *Infect Immun*, Vol.69, No.1, pp. 288-296, ***ISSN***: 0019-9567

Rigano, R., Profumo, E., Buttari, B., Teggi, A. &Siracusano, A. (1999a). Cytokine gene expression in peripheral blood mononuclear cells (PBMC) from patients with pharmacologically treated cystic echinococcosis. *Clin Exp Immunol*, Vol.118, No.1, pp. 95-101, ISSN: 1474-1741

Rigano, R., Profumo, E., Di Felice, G., Ortona, E., Teggi, A. &Siracusano, A. (1995a). In vitro production of cytokines by peripheral blood mononuclear cells from hydatid patients. *Clin Exp Immunol*, Vol.99, No.3, pp. 433-439, ISSN: 1474-1741

Rigano, R., Profumo, E., Ioppolo, S., Notargiacomo, S., Ortona, E., Teggi, A. &Siracusano, A. (1995b). Immunological markers indicating the effectiveness of pharmacological treatment in human hydatid disease. *Clin Exp Immunol*, Vol.102, No.2, pp. 281-285, ISSN: 1474-1741

Rigano, R., Profumo, E., Ioppolo, S., Notargiacomo, S., Teggi, A. &Siracusano, A. (1999b). Serum cytokine detection in the clinical follow up of patients with cystic echinococcosis. *Clin Exp Immunol*, Vol.115, No.3, pp. 503-507, ISSN: 1474-1741

Rigano, R., Profumo, E., Teggi, A. &Siracusano, A. (1996). Production of IL-5 and IL-6 by peripheral blood mononuclear cells (PBMC) from patients with *Echinococcus granulosus* infection. *Clin Exp Immunol*, Vol. 105, No.3, pp. 456-459, ISSN: 1474-1741

Ris, D. R., Hamel, K. L. &Mackle, Z. M. (1987). Use of two polysaccharide antigens in ELISA for the detection of antibodies to *Echinococcus granulosus* in sheep sera. *Res Vet Sci*, Vol.43, No.2, pp. 257-263, ISSN: 0034-5288

Romig, T. (2009). *Echinococcus multilocularis* in Europe--state of the art. *Vet Res Commun* Vol.33 No. Suppl 1: 31-34, ISSN:1573-7446

Rosenzvit, M. C., Camicia, F., Kamenetzky, L., Muzulin, P. M. &Gutierrez, A. M. (2006). Identification and intra-specific variability analysis of secreted and membrane-bound proteins from *Echinococcus granulosus*. *Parasitol Int*, Vol.55, Suppl: S63-67, ISSN: 1383-5769

Rott, M. B., Fernandez, V., Farias, S., Ceni, J., Ferreira, H. B., Haag, K. L. &Zaha, A. (2000). Comparative analysis of two different subunits of antigen B from *Echinococcus granulosus*: gene sequences, expression in Escherichia coli and serological evaluation. *Acta Trop*, Vol.75, No.3, pp. 331-340, ISSN: 0001-706X

Sadjjadi, S. M., Abidi, H., Sarkari, B., Izadpanah, A. &Kazemian, S. (2007). Evaluation of enzyme linked immunosorbent assay, utilizing native antigen B for serodiagnosis of human hydatidosis. *Iran J Immunol*, Vol.4, No.3, pp. 162-172, ISSN: 1735-1383

Sano, T., Smith, C. L. &Cantor, C. R. (1992). Immuno-PCR: very sensitive antigen detection by means of specific antibody-DNA conjugates. *Science*, Vol.258, No.5079, pp. 120-122, ISSN: 0036-8075

Schantz, P. M. (1988). Circulating antigen and antibody in hydatid disease. *N Engl J Med*, Vol.318, No.22, pp. 1469-1470, ISSN: 0028-4793

Shambesh, M. K., Craig, P. S., Wen, H., Rogan, M. T. &Paolillo, E. (1997). IgG1 and IgG4 serum antibody responses in asymptomatic and clinically expressed cystic echinococcosis patients. *Acta Trop*, Vol.64, No.1-2, pp. 53-63, ISSN: 0001-706X

Shepherd, J. C., Aitken, A. &McManus, D. P. (1991). A protein secreted in vivo by *Echinococcus granulosus* inhibits elastase activity and neutrophil chemotaxis. *Mol Biochem Parasitol*, Vol.44, No.1, pp. 81-90, ISSN: 0166-6851

Shepherd, J. C. &McManus, D. P. (1987). Specific and cross-reactive antigens of *Echinococcus granulosus* hydatid cyst fluid. *Mol Biochem Parasitol*, Vol.25, No.2, pp. 143-154, ISSN: 0166-6851

Siles-Lucas, M. M. &Gottstein, B. B. (2001). Molecular tools for the diagnosis of cystic and alveolar echinococcosis. *Trop Med Int Health*, Vol.6, No.6, pp. 463-475, ISSN: 1365-3156

Simsek, S. &Koroglu, E. (2004). Evaluation of enzyme-linked immunosorbent assay (ELISA) and enzyme-linked immunoelectrotransfer blot (EITB) for immunodiagnosis of hydatid diseases in sheep. *Acta Trop*, Vol.92, No.1, pp. 17-24, ISSN: 0001-706X

Siracusano, A., Buttari, B., Delunardo, F., Profumo, E., Margutti, P., Ortona, E., Rigano, R. &Teggi, A. (2004). Critical points in the immunodiagnosis of cystic echinococcosis in humans. *Parassitologia*, Vol.46, No.4, pp. 401-403, ISSN: 0048-2951

Sjolander, A., Guisantes, J. A., Torres-Rodriguez, J. M. &Schroder, H. (1989). The diagnosis of human hydatidosis by measurement of specific IgE antibody by enzyme immunoassay. *Scand J Infect Dis*, Vol.21, No.2, pp. 213-218, ISSN: 0036-5548

Speiser, F. (1980). Application of the enzyme-linked immunosorbent assay (ELISA) for the diagnosis of filariasis and echinococcosis. *Tropenmed Parasitol*, Vol.31, No.4, pp. 459-466, ISSN: 0303-4208

Sterla, S., Sato, H. &Nieto, A. (1999). *Echinococcus granulosus* human infection stimulates low avidity anticarbohydrate IgG2 and high avidity antipeptide IgG4 antibodies. *Parasite Immunol*, Vol.21, No.1, pp. 27-34, ISSN: 1365-3024

Tappe, D., Sako, Y., Itoh, S., Frosch, M., Gruner, B., Kern, P. &Ito, A. (2010). Immunoglobulin G subclass responses to recombinant Em18 in the follow-up of patients with alveolar echinococcosis in different clinical stages. *Clin Vaccine Immunol*, Vol.17, No.6, pp. 944-948, ISSN: 1556-679X

Tawfeek, G. M., Elwakil, H. S., El-Hoseiny, L., Thabet, H. S., Sarhan, R. M., Awad, N. S. &Anwar, W. A. (2011). Comparative analysis of the diagnostic performance of crude sheep hydatid cyst fluid, purified antigen B and its subunit (12 Kda), assessed by ELISA, in the diagnosis of human cystic echinococcosis. *Parasitol Res*, Vol.108, No.2, pp. 371-376, ISSN:0932-0113

Thompson, C. R. A. &McManus, D. P. (2001). Aetiology: parasites and life-cycles. In: *WHO/OIE Manual on Echinococcosis in Humans and Animals: a Public Health Problem of Global Concern*, J. Eckert, M. A. Gemmell, F.-X. Mesli and Z. S. Pawlowski (Eds.) World Organisation for Animal Health and World Health Organisation, ISBN 92-9044-522-X, Paris, France

Vacirca, D., Perdicchio, M., Campisi, E., Delunardo, F., Ortona, E., Margutti, P., Teggi, A., Gottstein, B. &Siracusano, A. (2011). Favourable prognostic value of antibodies anti-HSP20 in patients with cystic echinococcosis: a differential immunoproteomic approach. *Parasite Immunol*, Vol.33, No.3, pp. 193-198, ISSN: 1365-3024

van Doorn, H. R., Koelewijn, R., Hofwegen, H., Gilis, H., Wetsteyn, J. C., Wismans, P. J., Sarfati, C., Vervoort, T. &van Gool, T. (2007). Use of enzyme-linked immunosorbent assay and dipstick assay for detection of Strongyloides stercoralis infection in humans. *J Clin Microbiol*, Vol.45, No.2, pp. 438-442, ISSN: 1098-660X

Varela-Diaz, V. M., Coltorti, E. A., Prezioso, U., Lopez-Lemes, M. H., Guisantes, J. A. &Yarzabal, L. A. (1975a). Evaluation of three immunodiagnostic tests for human hydatid disease. *Am J Trop Med Hyg*, Vol.24, No.2, pp. 312-319, ISSN: 0002-9637

Varela-Diaz, V. M., Guisantes, J. A., Ricardes, M. I., Yarzabal, L. A. &Coltorti, E. A. (1975b). Evaluation of whole and purified hydatid fluid antigens in the diagnosis of human hydatidosis by the immunoelectrophoresis test. *Am J Trop Med Hyg*, Vol.24, No.2, pp. 298-303, ISSN: 0002-9637

Varela-Diaz, V. M., Lopez-Lemes, M. H., Prezioso, U., Coltorti, E. A. &Yarzabal, L. A. (1975c). Evaluation of four variants of the indirect hemagglutination test for human hydatidosis. *Am J Trop Med Hyg*, Vol.24, No.2, pp. 304-311, ISSN: 0002-9637

Verastegui, M., Moro, P., Guevara, A., Rodriguez, T., Miranda, E. &Gilman, R. H. (1992). Enzyme-linked immunoelectrotransfer blot test for diagnosis of human hydatid disease. *J Clin Microbiol*, Vol30, No.6, pp. 1557-1561, ISSN: 1098-660X

Virginio, V. G., Hernandez, A., Rott, M. B., Monteiro, K. M., Zandonai, A. F., Nieto, A., Zaha, A. &Ferreira, H. B. (2003). A set of recombinant antigens from *Echinococcus granulosus* with potential for use in the immunodiagnosis of human cystic hydatid disease. *Clin Exp Immunol*, Vol.132, No.2, pp. 309-315, ISSN: 1474-1741

Virginio, V. G., Taroco, L., Ramos, A. L., Ferreira, A. M., Zaha, A., Ferreira, H. B. &Hernandez, A. (2007). Effects of protoscoleces and AgB from *Echinococcus granulosus* on human neutrophils: possible implications on the parasite's immune evasion mechanisms. *Parasitol Res*, Vol.100, No.5, pp. 935-942, ISSN:0932-0113

Vogel, M., Gottstein, B., Muller, N. &Seebeck, T. (1988). Production of a recombinant antigen of *Echinococcus multilocularis* with high immunodiagnostic sensitivity and specificity. *Mol Biochem Parasitol*, Vol.31, No.2, pp. 117-125, ISSN: 0166-6851

Vuitton, D. A. (2003). The ambiguous role of immunity in echinococcosis: protection of the host or of the parasite? *Acta Trop*, Vol.85, No.2, pp. 119-132, ISSN: 0001-706X

Vuitton, D. A. (2004). Echinococcosis and allergy. *Clin Rev Allergy Immunol*, Vol.26, No.2, pp. 93-104, ISSN:1080-0549

Vuitton, D. A., Bresson-Hadni, S., Laroche, L., Kaiserlian, D., Guerret-Stocker, S., Bresson, J. L. &Gillet, M. (1989). Cellular immune response in *Echinococcus multilocularis* infection in humans. II. Natural killer cell activity and cell subpopulations in the blood and in the periparasitic granuloma of patients with alveolar echinococcosis. *Clin Exp Immunol*, Vol.78, No.1, pp.67-74, ISSN: 1474-1741

Wang, Y., He, T., Wen, X., Li, T., Waili, A., Zhang, W., Xu, X., Vuitton, D. A., Rogan, M. T., Wen, H. &Craig, P. S. (2006). Post-survey follow-up for human cystic echinococcosis in northwest China. *Acta Trop*, Vol.98, No.1, pp. 43-51, ISSN: 0001-706X

Wattal, C., Mohan, C. &Agarwal, S. C. (1988). Evaluation of specific immunoglobulin E by enzyme-linked immunosorbent assay in hydatid disease. *Int Arch Allergy Appl Immunol*, Vol.87, No.1, pp. 98-100, ISSN: 1018-2438

Wen, H. &Craig, P. S. (1994). Immunoglobulin G subclass responses in human cystic and alveolar echinococcosis. *Am J Trop Med Hyg*, Vol.51, No.6, pp. 741-748, ISSN: 0002-9637

Xiao, N., Mamuti, W., Yamasaki, H., Sako, Y., Nakao, M., Nakaya, K., Gottstein, B., Schantz, P. M., Lightowlers, M. W., Craig, P. S. &Ito, A. (2003). Evaluation of use of recombinant Em18 and affinity-purified Em18 for serological differentiation of alveolar echinococcosis from cystic echinococcosis and other parasitic infections. *J Clin Microbiol*, Vol.41, No.7, pp. 3351-3353, ISSN: 1098-660X

Yang, Y. R., Craig, P. S., Vuitton, D. A., Williams, G. M., Sun, T., Liu, T. X., Boufana, B., Giraudoux, P., Teng, J., Li, Y., Huang, L., Zhang, W., Jones, M. K. &McManus, D. P. (2008). Serological prevalence of echinococcosis and risk factors for infection among children in rural communities of southern Ningxia, China. *Trop Med Int Health*, Vol.13, No.8, pp.1086-1094, ISSN: 1365-3156

Yang, Y. R., Sun, T., Zhang, J. Z. &McManus, D. P. (2006). Molecular confirmation of a case of multiorgan cystic echinococcosis. *J Parasitol*, Vol.92, No.1, pp. 206-208, ISSN: 0022-3395

Yong, W. K., Heath, D. D. &Van Knapen, F. (1984). Comparison of cestode antigens in an enzyme-linked immunosorbent assay for the diagnosis of *Echinococcus granulosus*, *Taenia hydatigena* and T ovis infections in sheep. *Res Vet Sci*, Vol.36, No.1, pp. 24-31, *ISSN*: 0034-5288

Zarzosa, M. P., Orduna Domingo, A., Gutierrez, P., Alonso, P., Cuervo, M., Prado, A., Bratos, M. A., Garcia-Yuste, M., Ramos, G. &Rodriguez Torres, A. (1999). Evaluation of six serological tests in diagnosis and postoperative control of pulmonary hydatid disease patients. *Diagn Microbiol Infect Dis*, Vol.35, No.4, pp. 255-262, ISSN: 0732-8893

Zhang, S., Hue, S., Sene, D., Penfornis, A., Bresson-Hadni, S., Kantelip, B., Caillat-Zucman, S. &Vuitton, D. A. (2008a). Expression of major histocompatibility complex class I chain-related molecule A, NKG2D, and transforming growth factor-beta in the liver of humans with alveolar echinococcosis: new actors in the tolerance to parasites? *J Infect Dis*, Vol.197, No.9, pp. 1341-1349, ISSN: 0022-1899

Zhang, W., Li, J., Jones, M. K., Zhang, Z., Zhao, L., Blair, D. &McManus, D. P. (2010). The *Echinococcus granulosus* antigen B gene family comprises at least 10 unique genes in five subclasses which are differentially expressed. *PLoS Negl Trop Dis*, Vol.4, No.8, pp. e784, ISSN: 1935-2735

Zhang, W., Li, J. &McManus, D. P. (2003a). Concepts in immunology and diagnosis of hydatid disease. *Clin Microbiol Rev*, Vol.16, No.1, pp. 18-36, ISSN: 1098-6618

Zhang, W. &McManus, D. P. (2006). Recent advances in the immunology and diagnosis of echinococcosis. *FEMS Immunol Med Microbiol*, Vol.47, No.1, pp. 24-41, ISSN: 0928-8244

Zhang, W., Ross, A. G. &McManus, D. P. (2008b). Mechanisms of immunity in hydatid disease: implications for vaccine development. *J Immunol*, Vol.181, No.10, pp. 6679-6685, ISSN: 1550-6606

Zhang, W., You, H., Li, J., Zhang, Z., Turson, G., Aili, H., Wang, J. &McManus, D. P. (2003b). Immunoglobulin profiles in a murine intermediate host model of resistance for *Echinococcus granulosus* infection. *Parasite Immunol*, Vol.25, No.3, pp. 161-168, ISSN: 1365-3024

Zhang, W., You, H., Zhang, Z., Turson, G., Hasyet, A. &McManus, D. P. (2001). Further studies on an intermediate host murine model showing that a primary *Echinococcus granulosus* infection is protective against subsequent oncospheral challenge. *Parasitol Int*, Vol.50, No.4, pp. 279-283, ISSN: 1383-5769

Zhang, W. B., Li, J., Li, Q., Yang, D., Zhu, B., You, H., Jones, M. K., Duke, M. &McManus, D. P. (2007). Identification of a diagnostic antibody-binding region on the immunogenic protein EpC1 from *Echinococcus granulosus* and its application in population screening for cystic echinococcosis. *Clin Exp Immunol*, Vol.149, No.1, pp. 80-86, ISSN: 1474-1741

Zhang, W. B. &Zhao, D. Z. (1992). A comparison of calcification of hydatid cysts in sheep pasturred and post-feeded. *Chinese Journal of Veterinary Science & Technology*, Vol.22, No.9, pp. 28-29 (in Chinese), ISSN: 1673-4696

Part 4

Serological Diagnosis of Autoimmune Disease

9

Specific Coeliac Disease Antibodies and Microenteropathy

Mohammad Rostami Nejad and Mohammad Reza Zali
Celiac Disease Department,
Research Institute of Gastroenterology and Liver Disease,
Shahid Beheshti University of Medical Sciences, Tehran,
Iran

1. Introduction

Coeliac disease and dyspepsia are common conditions, and consume considerable resources in both investigation and treatment. In the last years, considerable changes in epidemiology of Coeliac disease (CD) have been observed. Recently several studies have been published on the prevalence and importance of CD in Iran and showed that 1 out of 166 healthy Iranian blood donors are affected by CD (1).

A marked increase in CD prevalence and incidence especially the gluten sensitivity with milder enteropathy has been reported, (1, 2) which can be at least partially explained by both the development of more sensitive serological tests and a high degree of disease suspicion (3, 4). The variability of in particular clinical (5) and histological aspects of CD may face the clinician often with uncertainty as some of the features might not quite fit in the diagnostic models in current guidelines (2).

Related malabsorptive symptoms, such as weight loss, diarrhea/steatorrhea and abdominal distension may not be necessarily observed in many CD (6). Atypical forms of CD have increased considerably (7) and the presence of dyspepsia as a unique symptom has been frequently attributed to CD (8). In classical CD with prominent malabsorptive features, dyspepsia may be one of the symptoms. It has been reported that the frequency of CD in people with dyspeptic complaints is 1.1-3%, which is two to nine times higher than in the general population around the world (6, 8-12). Anti-endomysial antibodies (EmA) were confirmed to be less sensitive than IgA tTG antibodies, although at present, human recombinant tissue transglutaminase (tTG) antibodies of IgA class are considered the most sensitive marker (8-11). Moreover, a new serological test that is, antibodies to deamidated gliadin peptides (DGP) - has been proposed as a screening test for CD, since many retrospective and perspective studies showed a very high diagnostic accuracy of this immune marker. AGA were the first serological markers routinely used for CD screening, allowing the identification of at-risk-patients for gluten-sensitive enteropathy, but at present their importance is only historical, since their predictive value is quite significantly lower than that of EmA and tTG antibodies. The sensitivity and specificity of tTG IgA is in the 93% to 97% range and, therefore, they represent the first-choice test for screening asymptomatic people like dyspeptic patients and for ruling out CD in symptomatic patients with a low pretest probability for CD (9).

In the present study we described the prevalence of gluten sensitive enteropathy in dyspeptic patients and compare the value of serology with histology in diagnosing CD.

2. Method

2.1 Patients and methods

Between November 2007 and October 2008, 5732 patients aged 15 years or more attended the Gastroenterology section of the Taleghani Hospital of Tehran, Iran. Four hundred and seven patients (193 men and 214 women) with dyspepsia were prospectively studied. The study was approved by the institutional ethics committees of Research center for gastroenterology and liver disease, Shahid Beheshti University of Medical sciences, and all participants signed a written informed consent.

Individuals were considered dyspeptic if they complained of persistent pain or uneasiness in the upper abdomen. Upper GI endoscopies were performed in these patients to diagnose common causes of dyspepsia including esophagitis, peptic ulcers, duodenitis and cancer. In addition, CD was identified by histological alterations characteristic of gluten sensitive enteropathy and by consistent CD serology.

Gastric biopsies were obtained for *H.pylori* detection and biopsies from the second part of the duodenum for histological processing. Histological diagnosis of CD was based on the presence of intraepithelial lymphocytes, crypts hyperplasia and/or villi atrophy. Biopsy results were classified as absence of CD (Marsh 0) or suggestive of CD (Marsh I to IIIc), according to Marsh criteria (13) and subsequently modified by Rostami et al. (14). The histological specimens were examined by two pathologists who did not know the endoscopic results and clinical history of the patients.

The optical density readings on enzyme-linked immunosorbent assay (ELISA) of 407 patients were analyzed for IgA class human antitissue transglutaminase (tTG) antibody and total serum IgA values according to the manufacturer's instructions (15). Determinations of IgA tTGA antibody were carried out using a commercially available kit (AESKULISA tTG, Germany). According to standardized methods, when a value higher than 15.0 U/ml was recorded, the result was considered positive. Total serum IgA values were measured by an immunoturbidometric assay (Pars Azmoon, Iran) and serum levels below 70 U/L were considered indicative of IgA deficiency. Those with IgA deficiency were tested with Immunoglobulin G (IgG) tTGG by an ELISA method, and using the commercially available kit (AESKULISA tTGG, Germany).

Serological data were correlated to the endoscopic results and to the histological pattern observed in the small intestine. All patients with confirmed CD diagnosis were treated with a gluten free diet and followed.

2.2 Statistical analysis

Statistical analysis was performed using SPSS software, version 13.5. Descriptive variables such as mean, median and standard deviation were determined. Chi-square ($\chi 2$) test was performed to find out the association between CD and risk factors.

3. Results

The mean age of the patients was 36.1 years. The gastroenterology symptoms in the subjects were: 78% abdominal pain, 70% bloating, 58% heart burn, 46% early satiety, 32% nausea, 32% flatulence, 31% weight loss and 22% anorexia. Recurrent abdominal pain, heart burn and bloating were present in 60%, 45% and 31% of the patients respectively.

H.pylori was detected in 90.5% cases. There were 26 cases with enteropathy (12 Marsh I, 4 Marsh II, 2 Marsh IIIa, 6 Marsh IIIb and 2 Marsh IIIc). Four of 407 dyspeptic patients were IgA deficient and all of them were negative for IgG tTG. Thirty three (8.1%) of the 407 patients tested had tTGA level more than 15 u/ml and considered as tTGA positive. Twenty three of 33 seropositive had normal small bowel mucosa.

The demographic, histologic and serologic characteristics of 33 patients with serology positive and 26 with abnormal histology are shown in table 1. In 10 of 33 tTGA positive patients CD was confirmed by histology analysis of the intestinal biopsy samples, giving a prevalence of CD of 2.45%. Five of these 10 coeliac patients were Marsh IIIa-c followed by 3 Marsh I and 2 Marsh II. The highest rate of histological abnormalites and of CD seropositivity was found in the age cathegories of 21-30 years and 10-20 years respectively.

			gender		GI symptoms									
subjects	no. of cases	Mean age	M	F	AP	AN	WL	NA	HB	ES	FL	BL	HP	CD
Abnormal histology patients	26	37.9	11	15	18	6	11	5	14	8	7	12	21	10
Seropositive patients	33	42.6	13	20	25	8	9	9	10	9	7	15	26	10

AP; abdominal discomfort, AN; anorexia, WL; weight loss, NA; nausea, HB; heart burn, Early satiety, FL; flatulence, BL; bloating, HP; *Helicobacter pylori*, CD; Coeliac disease

Table 1. Clinical and laboratory features of seropositive patients

4. Discussion

Dyspepsia is a highly prevalent and heterogeneous disorder (16). We know that damages in gluten sensitivity are not confined to the small intestine (17) and no every gluten sensitive patients develop severe mucosal small bowel abnormality. Several studies have demonstrated that continues exposure to gluten may damage the structure and function of the gastric mucosa in gluten-sensitive patients (18, 19). Other surveys indicate that approximately 20% of patients with dyspeptic symptoms have erosive esophagitis, 20% are estimated to have endoscopy-negative reflux disease, 10% have peptic ulcer, 2% have Barrett esophagus (20) and the results of the present study suggest that at least 2-3% coeliac disease with histology confirmation could be added to the list. However, the proportion of gluten related dyspepsia seems to be even higher (serology >8%) and hence gluten sensitivity might be a major etiology for dyspepsia.

The most important identifiable causes underlying dyspeptic symptoms in our study group were duodenitis (13%), gastritis (12%), esophagitis (9%) and peptic ulcer disease in 10% malignancies of the upper gastrointestinal tract were not found. Approximately 60% of patients with dyspepsia showed no abnormality in their mucosa but the majorities were positive for *H.pylori*.

A significant number (8%) of our cohort with dyspepsia had positive serology for CD. The large number with positive tTG in this study (in total 33 tTG positive which 23/33 had normal histology) would suggest that dyspepsia might represent a cardinal sign and a prevalent mod of presentation for gluten sensitivity. We found that anti-tTG IgA antibodies were highly specific but poorly sensitive for detecting severe villous atrophy in coeliac patients under a gluten free diet.

Immunoglobulin A (IgA), anti-endomysial antibodies (IgA EMA-ab) and IgA anti-tTG antibodies (IgA tTG-ab) are in close correlation in untreated as well as treated coeliac (fig 1) (21, 22). It is important to note that serology (EMA/tTGA) is a far more specific marker for atypical CD compared to microenteropathy (Marsh I-II) which seems to have a non-specific nature (23). In other word the specificity of serology for CD seems to be close to 99% in many studies (24). This is in contrast to histology that would have a non-specific value especially in cases with milder enteropathy (microscopic enteritis, Marsh 0-II). Obviously histology could represent the gold standard for CD diagnosis only in cases with severe mucosal abnormality (Marsh IIIa-c). Since tTG autoantibodies have a far higher specificity (>98-100%) for CD compared to a milder enteropathy, we might consider a higher prevalence (±8%) for CD in dyspeptic patients (25, 26). Testing for tTG antibodies is the cheapest and most accurate option, as the EMA method used to detect endomysial antibodies is subjective and uses expensive tissue of monkey oesophagus or umbilical cord as the substrate. When there is a low suspicion of CD, serological testing should be done as a high-specificity rule-in test, but when there is a high suspicion of CD, HLA typing as a high-sensitivity rule-out test would be useful. This strategy might be helpful in encouraging health professionals to use serology because the index of suspicion is generally low for atypical presentation. Perhaps performing HLA typing in seronegatives would give some more degree of reassurance in ruling it out.

Recent studies has clearly emphasized that, while IgA DGP antibodies do not add anything to the IgA tTG test, but IgG DGP antibodies are a relevant test for CD diagnosis and can identify the CD patients with IgA deficiency (27). In this CD subgroup, IgG DGP antibodies should be preferred to IgG tTG antibodies, whose positivity, as generally acknowledged, is fairly less specific and indicative of CD than that of IgG DGP antibodies (fig 1).

We are aware that there is no a single perfect test to diagnose CD in its own. Histological abnormalities were found in 26 (6.4%) of our patients. Despite high specificity of autoantibodies, this finding would provoke the discussion on seronegative cases and question the sensitivity of serological tests. Although, microenteropathy could be a result of any other intestinal disorder, from previous experience we learned those negative serological tests were less reliable in symptomatic cases presenting with a milder enteropathy (28- 30).

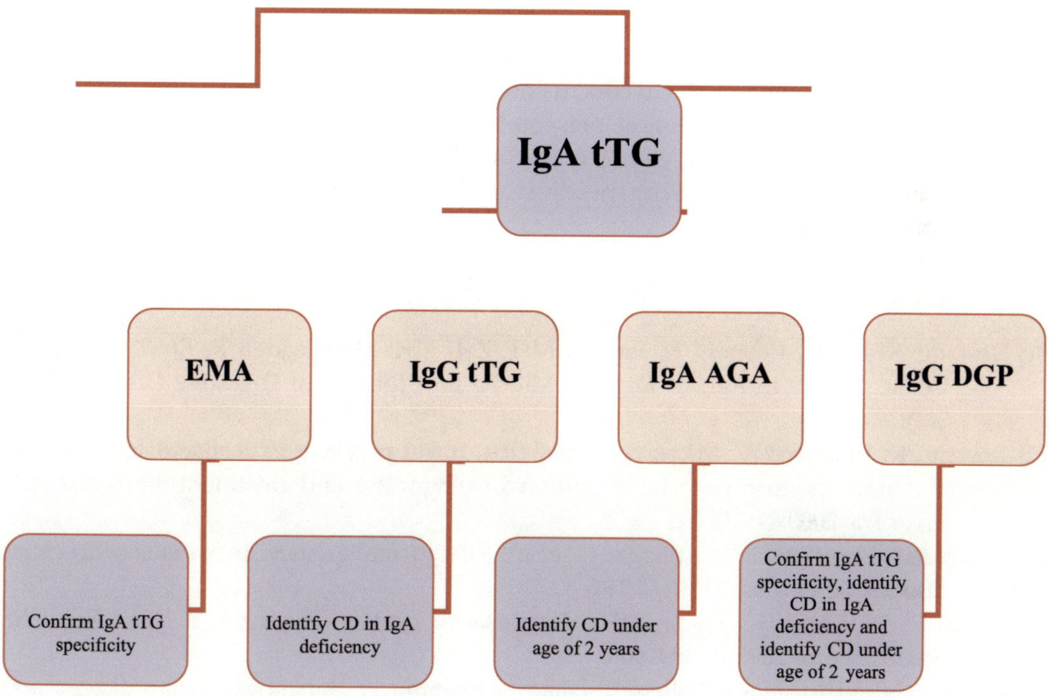

Fig. 1. Comparison between the present and new serological strategy for coeliac disease diagnosis

Based on this evidence if we believe that specificity of serology (tTGA) is beyond 98% and if we also believe that seronegative cases presenting with milder enteropathy exist, we might be able to recognize that an even higher proportion (>8%) of our CD patients might present with dyspepsia. In such cases in contrast to the high diagnostic value of severe enteropathy, microenteropathy obviously fails to represent the gold standard in diagnosis of gluten sensitivity as it is simply unreliable in its own. There is nothing against the fact that histology remains as an important component in diagnosis of GS but not as the gold standard at least in atypical cases with microenteropathy. Coeliac disease with flat mucosa based on which the gold standard was introduced >50 years ago is still a rare condition. It is time to recognize that for a good proportion of gluten sensitive cases histology is non-specific and hence the pathologist is unable to make the definite diagnosis in his own. Therefore, in conclusion, we suggest do not expect too much from histology and concentrate on clinical presentation and presence of autoantibodies as the diamond standard for diagnosis of CD. Future studies would be needed to assess whether dyspeptic patients presenting with positive antibodies and whatever histology would require gluten free diet?

5. Reference

[1] Rostami Nejad M, Rostami K, Emami MH, Zali MR, Malekzadeh R. Epidemiology of Celiac disease in Iran; A Review. Middle East Journal of Digestive Diseases 2011; 3(1): 74-77.

[2] Rostami K, Villanacci V. Microscopic enteritis: novel prospect in coeliac disease clinical and immuno-histogenesis. Evolution in diagnostic and treatment strategies. Dig Liver Dis 2009;41:245-52.

[3] Green PH, Fleischauer AT, Bhagat G, et al. Risk of malignancy in patients with celiac disease. Am J Med 2003;115:191–5.

[4] Green PH, Rostami K, Marsh MN. Diagnosis of coeliac disease. Best Pract Res Clin Gastroenterol 2005;19:389–400.

[5] Rostami Nejad M, Hogg-Kollars S, Ishaq S, Rostami K. Subclinical celiac disease and gluten sensitivity. Gastroenterol Hepatol Bed Bench. 2011;4(3): 102-108.

[6] Lima VM, Gandolfi L, Pires JAA, Pratesi R. Prevalence of Ccliac disease in dyspeptic patients. Arq Gastroenterol 2005; 42(3); 153-6

[7] Ciclitira PJ. AGA technical review on celiac sprue. American Gastroenterological Association practice guidelines. Gastroenterology 2001; 120:1526-40.

[8] Bardella MT,Minoli G, Ravizza D, Radaelli F, Velio P, Quatrini M, Bianchi PA, Conte D. Increased prevalence of Coeliac disease in patients with dyspepsia. Arch Intern Med 2000; 160:1489–1491

[9] Vivas S, Ruiz de Morales JM, Martinez J, Gonzalez MC, Martin S, Martin J, Cechini C, Olcoz JL. Human recombinant antitransglutaminase antibody testing is useful in the diagnosis of silent coeliac disease in a selected group of at-risk patients. Eur J Gastroenterol Hepatol 2003;15:479-83.

[10] Ozaslan E, Akkorlu S, Eskioglu E, Kayhan B. Prevalence of silent celiac disease in patients with dyspepsia. Dig Dis Sci. 2007; 52(3): 692-7

[11] Altintas E, Senli MS, Sezgin O. Prevalence of celiac disease among dyspeptic patients: A community-based case-control study. Turk J Gastroenterol. 2008; 19(2): 81-84.
[12] Giangreco E, D'Agate C, Barbera C, Puzzo L, Aprile G, Naso P, et al. Prevalence of Coeliac disease in adult patients with refractory functional dyspepsia: Value of routine duodenal biopsy. World J Gastroenterol. 2008; 14(45): 6948-53.
[13] Marsh MN. Gluten, major histocompatibility complex, and the small intestine. A molecular and immunobiological approach to the spectrum of gluten sensitivity. Gastroenterology 1992; 102: 330–354.
[14] Rostami K, Kerckhaert J, Tiemessen R, von Blomberg BM, Meijer JW, Mulder CJ. Sensitivity of antiendomysium and antigliadin antibodies in untreated Coeliac disease: disappointing in clinical practice. Am J Gastroenterol 1999; 94: 888-94.
[15] Rostami Nejad M, Rostami K, Pourhoseingholi MA et al. Atypical Presentation is Dominant and Typical for Coeliac Disease. J Gastrointestin Liver Dis. 2009; 18 (3): 285-291.
[16] Talley NJ, Zinsmeister AR, Schleck CD, Melton LJ, 3rd. Dyspepsia and dyspepsia subgroups: a population-based study. Gastroenterology 1992; 102:1259-68.
[17] Diamanti A, Maino C, Niveloni S, Pedreira S, Vazquez H, Smecuol E, Fiorini A, Cabanne A, Bartellini MA, Kogan Z, Valero J, Maurino E, Bai JC. Characterization of gastric mucosal lesions in patients with Coeliac disease: a prospective controlled study. Am J Gastroenterol 1999; 94:1313-9.
[18] Locke GR, 3rd, Murray JA, Zinsmeister AR, Melton LJ, 3rd, Talley NJ. Coeliac disease serology in irritable bowel syndrome and dyspepsia: a population-based case-control study. Mayo Clin Proc 2004;79:476-82.
[19] Bardella MT, Minoli G, Ravizza D, Radaelli F, Velio P, Quatrini M, Bianchi PA, onte D. Increased prevalence of Coeliac disease in patients with dyspepsia. Arch Intern Med 2000;160:1489-91.
[20] Moayyedi P, Talley NJ, Fennerty MB, Vakil N. Can the clinical history distinguish between organic and functional dyspepsia? Jama 2006;295:1566-76.
[21] Amin M, Eckhardt T, Kapitza S, et al. Correlation between tissue transglutaminase antibodies and antiendomysium antibodies as diagnostic markers of coeliac disease. Clin Chim Acta 1999;282:219–25.
[22] Sulkanen S, Halttunen T, Laurila K, et al. Tissue transglutaminase autoantibody enzyme-linked immunosorbent assay in detecting celiac disease. Gastroenterology 1998;115: 1322–8.
[23] Sbarbati A, Valletta E, Bertini M, Cipolli M, Morroni M, Pinelli L, Tato L. Gluten sensitivity and 'normal' histology: is the intestinal mucosa really normal? Dig Liver Dis 2003;35:768-73.
[24] Abrams JA, Diamond B, Rotterdam H, et al. Seronegative coeliac disease: increased prevalence with lesser degrees of villous atrophy. Dig Dis Sci. 2004;49: 546–50.
[25] Hill PG, Holmes GK. Coeliac disease: a biopsy is not always necessary for diagnosis. Aliment Pharmacol Ther 2008;27:572-7.
[26] Ludvigsson JF, Brandt L, Montgomery SM. Symptoms and signs in individuals with serology positive for Coeliac disease but normal mucosa. BMC Gastroenterol 2009;9:57.

[27] Volta U, Granito A, Parisi C, Fabbri A, Fiorini E, Piscaglia M, et al. Deamidated gliadin peptide antibodies as a routine test for Coeliac disease: a prospective analysis. J Clin Gastroenterol. 2010; 44(3):186-90.

[28] Diamanti A, Maino C, Niveloni S, Pedreira S, Vazquez H, Smecuol E, Fiorini A, Cabanne A, Bartellini MA, Kogan Z, Valero J, Maurino E, Bai JC. Characterization of gastric mucosal lesions in patients with celiac disease: a prospective controlled study. Am J Gastroenterol 1999;94:1313-9.

[29] Locke GR, Murray JA, Zinsmeister AR, Melton LJ, Talley NJ. Coeliac disease serology in irritable bowel syndrome and dyspepsia: a population-based case-control study. Mayo Clin Proc 2004;79:476-82.

[30] Tack J, Lee KJ. Pathophysiology and treatment of functional dyspepsia. J Clin Gastroenterol 2005;39:S211-6.